Management of Restless Legs Syndrome

Second Edition

Hochang B. Lee, MD
Associate Professor of Psychiatry
Yale University School of Medicine

Mark J. Buchfuhrer, MD
Consulting Assistant Professor,
Department of Sleep Medicine
Stanford University School of Medicine
Medical Director, SleepMed of Cypress, California

Richard Allen, PhD
Associate Professor, Department of Neurology
Johns Hopkins University

Wayne A. Hening, MD
1945–2008

PROFESSIONAL
COMMUNICATIONS, INC.

Professional Communications, Inc.

A Medical Publishing & Communications Company

400 Center Bay Drive	PO Box 10
West Islip, NY 11795	Caddo, OK 74729-0010
(t) 631/661-2852	(t) 580/745-9838
(f) 631/661-2167	(f) 580/745-9837

For orders only, please call
1-800-337-9838

or visit our Web site at
www.pcibooks.com

ISBN: 978-1-932610-88-8

Printed in the United States of America

DISCLAIMER

The opinions expressed in this publication reflect those of the authors. However, the authors make no warranty regarding the contents of the publication. The protocols described herein are general and may not apply to a specific patient. Any product mentioned in this publication should be taken in accordance with the prescribing information provided by the manufacturer.

This text is printed on recycled paper.

DEDICATION

To Wayne, whose compassion for RLS patients inspired his colleagues and trainees alike to "open a window into a deeper world" of this mysterious condition. We all miss Wayne, a wonderful friend, clinician, and teacher of all things related to RLS.

— **HBL, MJB, RA**

To Rebecca, my daughter, whose birth was celebrated by Wayne and me as we developed the RLS in Baltimore Epidemiologic Catchment Area (RiBECA) Study together.

— **HBL**

ACKNOWLEDGMENT

I would like to acknowledge the assistance of
Jacqueline Vachon, MS, LPC.
— **HBL**

TABLE OF CONTENTS

TABLES

FIGURES

1   What Is RLS (or WED)?

RLS (or WED) is a Neurological Sensorimotor Disorder

The restless legs syndrome (RLS), named by Karl Ekbom,[1] has a name that suggests some minor irritation and, for some who have a mild case, that is all it is. However, the name is misleading when applied to those who have a more severe condition. They experience an almost overwhelming need to move and a discomfort that can be so excruciating that it can be called "torture" (as Thomas Willis suggested describing a case in the 17th century[2]). It also minimizes the scope of the disorder; severe patients can have arm involvement as well and sometimes discomfort in the trunk, pelvis, and even in the face. Given these problems with the name restless legs, the professional and patient associations have recently advocated a more appropriate name of Willis-Ekbom Disease (WED). This avoids focusing on any one aspect of the disease and recognizes the first doctors to best describe the disease in the medical literature. WED is becoming more accepted in the literature and will be used in this book interchangeably with RLS.

RLS produces both sensory and motor symptoms. The primary symptom is a strange feeling of an urge or strong need to move that is focused on one or both legs and sometimes other parts of the body. This sense of a need to move is exacerbated or even started by rest. RLS patients are intolerant of rest, particularly in the evening or night when the symptoms become worse. This primary symptom of an urge to move will often feel very uncomfortable and even painful, and it is often associated with other uncomfortable sensations usually also localized to the legs (**Table 1.1**) or

TABLE 1.1 — Terms Often Used by Patients to Describe Their RLS Symptoms

- Creepy, crawly
- Insects crawling or worms wiggling in legs
- Itchy bones
- Soda in veins
- Achy pain
- Heebie-jeebies
- The "got to moves"
- The fidgets
- Electric shock feeling
- Crampy feeling

other affected body parts. In addition to these sensory symptoms, RLS also has motor components that are both voluntary and involuntary. The voluntary part is the response of the patients to their discomfort or need to move. The movement relieves the RLS symptoms. There is no specific form to these voluntary movements, although walking is the most common. RLS patients may also stretch, bend, kick, or bicycle in order to obtain relief. They learn to use the movements that most effectively relieve their discomfort in a given situation.

The involuntary part is the presence of repetitive movements that patients cannot control, referred to as periodic limb movements (PLM). These most often are present in sleep (PLM in sleep or PLMS [**Table 1.2**]) but can also occur when one is awake. For some patients, these uncontrolled jerking movements are themselves the most distressing symptom they experience. They typically recur every 10 to 40 seconds and are sometimes associated with a surge of sensory discomfort. Some RLS patients, however, do not have PLM. Moreover the PLMS appears to reflect a brain activation producing episodic arousals from sleep. The PLMS do not cause the arousal, rather the reverse. These frequent often disturbing arousal events cause the PLM. Some medications reducing the PLMS do not significantly reduce these episodic arousals.

TABLE 1.2 — Abbreviations Associated With RLS

PLM	Periodic Limb Movement(s)—One or more movements that meet the criteria for relatively stereotyped repetitive periodic movements (criteria including number in series, period, duration, amplitude), but not restricted to the sleep state.
PLMS	Periodic Limb Movement(s) in Sleep—One or more PLM occurring in sleep. Usually used as the plural to refer to all of such movements restricted to sleep that occur during a night's study or to the condition of having such movements, generally (eg, "The patient has PLMS").
PLMW	Periodic Limb Movement(s) in Wake—One or more PLM occurring during wake.
PLMD	Periodic Limb Movement Disorder—A medical disorder with symptoms indicative of sleep disturbance. This diagnosis requires documentation of some minimum number or frequency of PLM plus some related clinical complaint such as daytime sleepiness that cannot be accounted for by another disorder. Patients with RLS cannot have PLMD.
PLMI	Periodic Limb Movement Index—Number of PLM per hour.
PLMAI	Periodic Limb Movement Arousal Index—Number of PLMS per hour of sleep associated with an arousal on polysomnography. If enumerated, one or more such movements are PLMA and their sum can be abbreviated as #PLMA.

Thus increased arousals in sleep and waking are also a symptom of RLS, causing significant reduction in total sleep time. The PLMS provide a convenient measure of these arousal events. It is also important to appreciate that while PLMS usually occur with RLS, many people with PLMS do not have RLS. Thus, the sensory symptoms are required to identify RLS; PLMS alone do not suffice.

Is RLS (or WED) a New Disorder?

For some who are just becoming aware of RLS, it may seem like a new disorder. Until the last couple of decades, RLS remained an obscure diagnosis that was rarely taught and little studied. This, like many other sleep-related disorders, is not a new disease. Many sleep-related disorders were ignored or minimized until the development of sleep medicine in the middle of the 20th century. Like sleep apnea or rapid eye movement (REM) behavior disorder, conditions that sound like restless legs were described in several literary mentions, eg, Greek philosopher Chrysippus, who could not remain at rest during evening discussions. Willis in the later part of the 17th century may have been the first to describe a case in the medical literature:

> "…whilst they would indulge sleep, in their beds, immediately follow leapings up of the Tendons, in their Arms and Legs, with Cramps, and such unquietness and flying about of their members, that the sick can no more sleep, than those on the Rack." *(translated from Latin)*[3]

The rack, of course, was a premodern torture device that stretched the body until it began to break. What lends greater likelihood to this description being one of RLS was Willis' treatment—laudanum, an opioid preparation that is a member of one class of drugs that have been used quite successfully to treat RLS (see *Chapter 9*).

The first truly comprehensive description of RLS was Ekbom's monograph[1] published in 1945, supplemented by his later papers. Ekbom appreciated that RLS is provoked by rest and that patients move in many various ways to relieve their discomfort. He understood that symptoms most likely occurred at night and that sleep could be sorely disrupted. He recognized a familial tendency and such causes as iron deficiency or pregnancy. He suggested that this was likely to be a common condition and that RLS could be readily diagnosed by a careful, pertinent clinical interview.

RLS (or WED) Is a Common Condition

Ekbom found that 5% of his clinic patients could be diagnosed with RLS (or WED). While Ekbom described the symptoms of RLS, a consensus clinical definition was first promulgated by the International RLS Study Group (IRLSSG) in 1995.[4] This was updated and clarified in a consensus meeting of the IRLSSG at the National Institute of Health in Washington DC[5] and the most recent update of these criteria are available on the IRLSSG web site at www. IRLSSG.org. This 2003 consensus on four essential clinical features of RLS (see *Chapter 2*) led to more reliable epidemiologic studies, which confirmed that RLS is common—somewhere between 5% and 10% of adults in the community indicate that they experience these four features.[6,7] Most of the previous large scale studies that have used the 2003 clinical definition have been conducted in Europe and North America. The frequency of RLS is less certain in other regions, such as Asia, but appears to occur to some degree in all populations studied.

It is also important to define a group of those with RLS symptoms who are disturbed by the condition and merit medical attention. The REST epidemiologic studies delineated such a group by combining frequency of symptoms with a measure of impact: the degree to which individuals were bothered by the symptoms.[6]

Those who had symptoms at least twice a week and were bothered at least moderately by symptoms when they occurred were designated as RLS sufferers. They were estimated to make up approximately 2.7% of the adult population. A recent study using actual physician diagnoses has confirmed that 2% to 3% of the adult population in a primary care practice suffers from RLS.[8] While less common in children, such clinically significant RLS is not rare; about 1% of teenagers are RLS sufferers and even 0.5% of younger children.[9] These numbers are such that every physician will come into contact with patients who have RLS that merits intervention; some physicians—particularly those in specialties dealing with secondary RLS (due to pregnancy, iron deficiency, kidney failure, neuropathy, diabetes, rheumatoid arthritis)—are likely to see many such patients. Unfortunately, although common with significant morbidity and treatable, it remains even today often ignored or minimized.

RLS (or WED) Untreated Causes Significant Morbidity and a Major Cost to Our Society

The symptoms of RLS are themselves bothersome; patients dislike having them and strive to avoid them. However, this often requires avoiding personally meaningful activities that might provoke symptoms: lectures, conferences, desk work, theater, travel, dinner parties, and so on. Some patients cannot sit and watch TV or even sit and work on a computer. Virginia Wilson, a patient advocate who wrote the first patient's perspective book on RLS for the general public,[10] had to prepare her manuscript while standing up, continually moving her feet to avoid her RLS. Other patients have had to quit their chosen occupations: Ekbom, for instance, mentions a truck driver who had symptoms whenever driving and had to abandon that line of work. A general population survey in the United States found that severe primary RLS such as these cases had a 50% reduction in work productivity and moderate-to-severe RLS had a 20% reduction equivalent to losing work one day a week or more.[11] This creates a large social cost to not providing effective treatment for RLS.

A major problem in RLS patients and the complaint that historically has most led patients to seek medical attention for their symptoms is the disruption of sleep. Because of their symptoms, they may find it difficult to get to sleep. When they awaken, perhaps caused by intermittent arousals, they may have a reactivation of their symptoms. Patients with severe RLS/ WED may experience only a few hours of fragmented sleep in the course of the night—a degree of sleep deprivation equal to, if not exceeding, that of any other sleep disorder.[12]

Their sleep problems then become the basis for further morbidities.[13] These problems include fatigue, difficulty concentrating, depressed mood, and excessive daytime sleepiness. Thinking and judgment can be impaired. Studies have now shown that RLS patients are more likely to have anxiety disorders and depression, even compared with those with other chronic disorders.[14] The RLS patients were also more likely to attribute their mood disorders to their symptoms than were the controls. Recent studies have even suggested that RLS may be associated with physical disorders, such as hypertension and cardiovascular disease.[15] While these cross-sectional studies do not establish RLS as the cause of the psychiatric and medical disorders, they do raise the possibility and underline the importance of the condition.

In summary, RLS is not a trivial disease. While those with rarely occurring symptoms can easily adapt to their condition, the 2% to 3% of adults with significant disease represent an important clinical challenge. It is clearly not "disease mongering" to recommend the appropriate diagnosis and treatment of such patients—a population that too often went without diagnosis or appropriate treatment in the past.[16] To vividly illustrate the historical frustration and lack of treatment of these patients, it is instructive to read the many personal testimonials in a book by Robert Yoakum, another RLS sufferer.[17] For many patients with severe RLS, it is the worst problem of their lives.

The aim of this book is to provide the tools necessary to accurately diagnose and appropriately treat RLS patients. The bulk of the text will be devoted to this aim. For background, we will provide some information about the epidemiology, genetics, and pathophysiology of the condition. We will also provide information about the range of RLS patients—both idiopathic and secondary—that may be encountered in different practices and the special requirements for their treatment. Our emphasis will be on the basics of managing RLS (or WED), but we will include enough information to facilitate the management of the more difficult or complicated patient.

REFERENCES

1. Ekbom KA. Restless legs: a clinical study. *Acta Med Scand Supplementum*. 1945;158(suppl):1-122.

2. Willis T. *De Animae Brutorum*. London: Wells and Scott; 1672.

3. Willis T. *Two Discourses Concerning the Soul of Brutes*. London, England: Dring, Harper, and Leigh; 1683.

4. Walters AS. Toward a better definition of the restless legs syndrome. The International Restless Legs Syndrome Study Group. *Mov Disord*. 1995;10(5):634-642.

5. Allen RP, Picchietti D, Hening WA, Trenkwalder C, Walters AS, Montplaisi J; Restless Legs Syndrome Diagnosis and Epidemiology workshop at the National Institutes of Health; International Restless Legs Syndrome Study Group. Restless legs syndrome: diagnostic criteria, special considerations, and epidemiology. A report from the restless legs syndrome diagnosis and epidemiology workshop at the National Institutes of Health. *Sleep Med*. 2003;4(2):101-119.

6. Berger K, Luedemann J, Trenkwalder C, John U, Kessler C. Sex and the risk of restless legs syndrome in the general population. *Arch Intern Med*. 2004;164(2):196-202.

7. Allen RP, Walters AS, Montplaisir J, et al. Restless legs syndrome prevalence and impact: REST general population study. *Arch Intern Med*. 2005;165(11):1286-1292.

8. Allen RP, Stillman P, Myers AJ. Physician-diagnosed restless legs syndrome in a large sample of primary medical care patients in western Europe: Prevalence and characteristics. *Sleep Med*. 2010;11(1):31-37.

9. Picchietti D, Allen RP, Walters AS, Davidson JE, Myers A, Ferini-Strambi L. Restless legs syndrome: prevalence and impact in children and adolescents—the Peds REST study. *Pediatrics*. 2007;120(2):253-266.

10. Wilson VN, Buchholz D, Walters AS. *Sleep Thief: Restless Legs Syndrome*. Orange Park, FL: Galaxy Books; 1996.

11. Allen RP, Bharmal M, Calloway M. Prevalence and disease burden of primary restless legs syndrome: results of a general population survey in the United States. *Mov Disord*. 2011; 26(1):114-120.

12. Allen RP, Earley CJ. Restless legs syndrome: a review of clinical and pathophysiologic features. *J Clin Neurophysiol*. 2001;18(2):128-147.

19

13. Kushida CA, Allen RP, Atkinson MJ. Modeling the causal relationships between symptoms associated with restless legs syndrome and the patient-reported impact of RLS. *Sleep Med*. 2004;5(5):485-488.

14. Winkelmann J, Prager M, Lieb R, et al. "Anxietas tibiarum." Depression and anxiety disorders in patients with restless legs syndrome. *J Neurol*. 2005;252(1):67-71.

15. Winkelman JW, Finn L, Young T. Prevalence and correlates of restless legs syndrome symptoms in the Wisconsin Sleep Cohort. *Sleep Med*. 2006;7(7):545-552.

16. Hening W, Walters AS, Allen RP, Montplaisir J, Myers A, Ferini-Strambi L. Impact, diagnosis and treatment of restless legs syndrome (RLS) in a primary care population: the REST (RLS epidemiology, symptoms, and treatment) primary care study. *Sleep Med*. 2004;5(3):237-246.

17. Yoakum R. *Restless Legs Syndrome: Relief and Hope for Sleepless Victims of a Hidden Epidemic*. New York, NY: Fireside; 2006.

2

Diagnosis of RLS and Mimics

Diagnosis of RLS

■ **The 2011 Revised IRLSSG Diagnostic Criteria for RLS and the Five Diagnostic Features: URGES**

In 2011, the IRLSSG announced the revised diagnostic criteria (http://irlssg.org/diagnostic-criteria) for RLS that replaces the 2002 IRLSSG-NIH consensus diagnostic criteria (or often referred as "NIH RLS criteria").[1,2] The 2002 NIH RLS diagnostic criteria had previously emphasized the four following essential diagnostic features only: 1) Urge to move the legs; 2) Rest induced the urges; 3) Symptoms gets better with activity; and 4) evenings and nights are worse due to ubiquitously diurnal variation of RLS symptoms. However, several studies, most notably by the late Wayne Henning, illustrated that a variety of conditions, including cramps, positional discomfort, and local leg pathology, can often satisfy all four features of the 2002 NIH RLS diagnostic criteria and thereby "mimic" RLS.[3] In order to improve the validity of RLS diagnosis, the 2011 revised diagnostic criteria add the fifth criterion that emphasizes importance of evaluation for "mimics" and consideration for differential diagnoses before making a firm diagnosis of RLS.

The diagnosis of RLS is a clinical diagnosis. There is no specific test to order, and no pathognomic findings on exam or in the laboratory. The art and challenge of clinical diagnosis for RLS lies in its diurnal nature and the subjectivity of its symptoms. A clinician evaluating a patient during daytime cannot observe the late evening RLS symptoms. Therefore, an RLS diagnosis is based on complex interaction between the patient with the "hard to describe feelings" and the expert clinician who confirms the diagnostic features of RLS while considering differential diagnoses and excluding RLS mimics.

There are five diagnostic features that must be present to make a definite diagnosis of RLS (**Table 2.1**). These can be remembered under the acronym **URGES** (**Table 2.2**). This acronym emphasizes the key symptom of RLS: an urge to move the legs, usually accompanied or caused by unpleasant, uncomfortable sensations in the legs. The next three diagnostic features indicate those situations that provoke or ameliorate the urge (or akathisia). The final or fifth criterion emphasizes the need for consideration for potential "mimics" and differential diagnoses.

1. Urge to Move the Legs

The urge or need to move in RLS is a specific sensation that is usually localized to the legs. The most common exasperated expression of patients when asked about this symptom is "I just have to move. I can't keep still." This is not some generalized anxiety or unsettled feeling but a specific feeling in the legs. Patients can point to the location of their symptoms. The urge to move is also not an observation or judgment; the patient must experience the urge. There are people who tap their feet or shake their legs inadvertently. They are unconscious of their habitual movement until their attention is called to it and do not and cannot describe an actual need to move. This is not RLS. Most patients with clinically significant RLS say that when they have the urge to move, they cannot resist moving their legs.

Most patients can also describe an unpleasant sensation in the legs, although a small minority of patients denies an unpleasant sensation and only describes an isolated urge to move. Those who report sensations may attribute their need to move to this symptom, which may be described in a wide variety of ways (**Table 1.1**). Almost invariably, the sensation will be described using negative terms. Typically, the sensation is experienced within the limb, in the muscles, or in bones. It is less likely to be felt in the joints or in the feet, although such a distribution does occur. The most common location is between knee and ankle, although symptoms frequently occur above the knee. In most patients, the feeling is bilateral, although often one leg is more involved than the other. Rarely, the feeling is unilateral. The site and the laterality of the symptoms may vary from night to night. On rare occasions, few patients have reported that their legs alternate with only a single leg symptomatic on a given night. It is uncommon for the feeling to be localized to the skin surface. The area of involvement is usually nontender; rubbing or massaging the skin over the sensation tends to bring relief rather than provoking additional discomfort

The primary symptom of RLS is a persistent feeling that will last for a sustained period until the patient moves. It is not a brief or fleeting sensation, and it is not specifically positional. It is rarely, and very briefly if it is, relieved by a change of posture. Sustained relief from this often irresistible urge requires continuous movement. Some patients may say that their RLS symptoms are brief. However, if asked to specify the duration of moving before they can have relief without movements, they report many minutes or even hours before the urge to move no longer persists.

Patients with severe RLS frequently experience their RLS symptoms on other parts of body beside the legs. Most commonly, symptoms are felt in the arms.[4] Less commonly, the hips, trunk, shoulders, genitals, or anal region may be involved. The patient will describe the sensation in the extended area as being the same or very similar to the symptoms in their legs, and it will be generally characterized by the same akathisia-like features (diagnostic criteria 2 to 4). Typically, a patient with severe RLS would report that upper limb symptoms are experienced less frequently than those in the legs and begin later in the course of the disorder. It is rare for the RLS symptoms to develop in other body parts prior to develop in leg. Also, it is extremely rare

TABLE 2.1 — The Five Diagnostic Features of RLS

- An urge to move the legs usually but not always accompanied by or felt to be caused by uncomfortable and unpleasant sensations in the legs.[a,b]
- The urge to move the legs and any accompanying unpleasant sensations begin or worsen during periods of rest or inactivity such as lying down or sitting.
- The urge to move the legs and any accompanying unpleasant sensations are partially or totally relieved by movement, such as walking or stretching, at least as long as the activity continues.[c]
- The urge to move the legs and any accompanying unpleasant sensations during rest or inactivity only occur or are worse in the evening or night than during the day.[d]
- The occurrence of the above features are not solely accounted for as symptoms primary to another medical or a behavioral condition (eg, myalgia, venous stasis, leg edema, arthritis, leg cramps, positional discomfort, habitual foot tapping.)[e]

Specifiers for Clinical Course of RLS[f]
- Chronic-persistent RLS: Symptoms when not treated would occur on average at least twice weekly for the past year.
- Intermittent RLS: symptoms when not treated would occur on average < 2/week for the past year, with at least 5 lifetime events.

Specifier for Clinical Significance for RLS
- The symptoms of RLS cause significant distress or impairment in social, occupational, educational, or other important areas of functioning by the impact on sleep, energy/vitality, daily activities, behavior, cognition, or mood

[a] Sometimes the urge to move the legs is present without the uncomfortable sensations and sometimes the arms or other parts of the body are involved in addition to the legs.
[b] For children, the description of these symptoms should be in the child's own words.
[c] When symptoms are very severe, relief by activity may not be noticeable but must have been previously present.

Continued

TABLE 2.1 — *Continued*

^d When symptoms are very severe, the worsening in the evening or night may not be noticeable but must have been previously present.

^e These conditions, often referred to as "RLS mimics," have been commonly confused with RLS, particularly in surveys, because they produce symptoms that meet or at least come very close to meeting all of the above criteria. The list here gives some examples that have been noted as particularly significant in epidemiologic studies and clinical practice. RLS may also occur with any of these conditions, but the RLS symptoms will then be more in degree, conditions of expression, or character than those usually occurring as part of the other condition.

^f The clinical course criteria do not apply either for pediatric cases or for some special cases of provoked RLS such as pregnancy or drug-induced RLS where the frequency may be high but limited to duration of the provocative condition.

TABLE 2.2 — **URGES: The Five Clinical Features of RLS**

- **U**rge to move the legs
- **R**est induced
- **G**ets better with activity
- **E**vening and night worse
- **S**olely not accounted by another medical or behavioral conditions

---

to have RLS symptoms in other body parts beside legs to be the sole or major manifestation of RLS.

The majority of those with RLS symptoms differentiate their symptoms from pain; the symptoms are definitely unpleasant, usually not painful. However, pain is a common descriptor for those with more frequent and severe symptoms, reaching the majority in at least one case series.[5] In our experience, almost all patients who say their symptoms are painful liken them to an ache. Almost all of them will differentiate this pain-like RLS symptom from a muscle cramp, which nearly everyone has experienced more or less. A muscle spasm provides a pain of a different order and intensity—a sharp, severe pain as opposed to the ache of RLS symptoms.

2. Rest Induced

RLS symptoms are evoked by rest. Patients are readily aware that if they sit or lie down, they will develop symptoms after a period of time. The rapidity of symptom onset is one measure of the severity of RLS symptoms. If symptoms begin while a patient is active, this is very unlikely to be caused by RLS. However, patients with severe RLS may experience symptoms while standing quietly and symptoms may persist as they begin to move around.

Rest is a quiescent state; it implies both lack of motor activity and a general easing of alertness. It should not be position dependent. For most patients, lying is more likely to produce symptoms than sitting upright. In the Johns Hopkins family study, a diagnosis of definite RLS required that the person have more symptoms when lying down than when upright.[6] There does seem, however, to be a group of younger individuals who experience RLS only when sitting; at bed time, they can rapidly fall asleep before they develop any RLS symptoms. Such individuals usually have clinically insignificant RLS. A more persistent state of rest (eg, during theater, dinner parties, long distance trip, etc) can cause symptoms even during daytime although they tend to be uncommon.

Particularly difficult for RLS patients is a state of confinement. An airplane flight is a classic example of spatial confinement, especially in a seat with restricted room and blocked access to the aisle. RLS patients generally indicate that they are fearful of a situation in which they were unable to move freely. This leads to great mental stress and panic, and doing whatever movement to relief RLS symptoms in the confined space. Studies have shown that when patients are required to remain at rest, RLS symptoms will increase in the first hour at any time of day.[7,8]

3. Relieved by Movement

Patients with RLS readily discover that movement can relieve their symptoms. This relief generally lasts as long as the movement continues. The most typical movement is walking, but various other movements can be undertaken, such as flexing and extending the legs, stretching the legs, pumping the legs, shaking the legs, or moving the trunk or arms. They are all aimed to relieve the leg discomfort. Relief is usually felt quickly; many patients report that they feel better almost immediately after they begin to move. For some patients, however, it takes more time for relief. This is particularly true of patients with very severe RLS. Elderly patients with compromised mobility may find that it is difficult for them to achieve the level of movement vigorous enough to provide complete relief for RLS symptoms.

Two other forms of activity provide relief. One is mental—an exciting or stimulating activity that may not require much actual movement, such as game playing, watching a stimulating movie, or even arguing, can provide relief. The other is sensory; patients may report that massage, striking the leg, applying pressure, or rubbing on lotion may provide relief.

If asked, patients with severe RLS may report that they do not obtain relief with movement, but often they mean that movement does not provide continuing relief: once they sit or lie back down, they find that the discomfort quickly returns. However, during the period of movement, they do obtain relief. In a patient who can walk normally, relief should persist as long as the movement continues. Moreover, RLS symptoms should never begin during active movement.

4. Evening or Night Worse

Most patients indicate that their symptoms are worse at night or only occur at night. The exceptions are those patients with very severe RLS who may have symptoms at any time of the day with enough inactivity or those with mild RLS who only experience symptoms when they remain at rest for a prolonged period of time. However, the peak time period for the most severe RLS symptoms can vary considerably among patients from the evening, to bedtime, or even later in the night. While some RLS patients have symptoms in one of these periods, patients with more severe RLS may have symptoms that begin in the evening or even earlier in the day and persist through much of the night. They may have difficulty falling asleep and staying asleep because of their symptoms.

Previously, clinicians assumed that RLS symptoms were worse in the evening because most people rest in the evening. In other words, the fourth diagnostic criterion ("evening and night worse") was only an epiphenomenon of the second criterion (rest induced). However, several studies have now established that the symptoms of RLS follow a true circadian pattern, with the peak severity of RLS symptoms occurring during the early part of the night (23:00 to 4:00) and a protected period early in the day (9:00 to 13:00).[9,10] By having patients follow a constant routine and requiring multiple periods of rest (using a suggested immobilization test [**Table 2.3**]), it was possible to show that the circadian alteration of symptoms was not caused by rest alone but also depended on time of day. Symptom

TABLE 2.3 — Procedure for Suggested Immobilization Test

- Subject sits with legs outstretched, usually on a bed
- Subject is instructed not to move unless it is absolutely necessary
- No diverting activity is permitted (no television, reading, radio, talking)
- One or more leg symptoms are monitored by questionnaire or visual analogue scale (VAS) at intervals of 5 to 15 minutes
- Leg movements (or activity) are measured by electromyelogram (EMG) on the tibialis anterior or actigraphy of the legs
- The subject is monitored visually or by sleep recording to ensure that sleep does not occur

severity also did not depend on the timing of sleep deprivation since RLS symptoms were also reduced during the protected period after a night of sleep deprivation. Symptoms occurred during the falling phase of core body temperature and began to dissipate as core temperature rose in the period before waking (**Figure 2.1**).[9,10] One study measured another circadian marker, melatonin, which begins to rise within a few hours of normal bedtime and remains elevated during the night, decreasing as the sleep period ends.[11] In that study, the severity RLS symptoms matched the period of elevated melatonin. The relationship of RLS symptoms to the overall circadian rhythm controlled by the suprachiasmatic nucleus is less clear. Although one research group has suggested that melatonin, which suppresses dopamine, may be responsible for the nocturnal peak of RLS symptoms,[11] this potential link remains unproven. One manifestation of the circadian accentuation of RLS symptoms is the more rapid development of RLS symptoms during the late evening and night.[7,8]

A common finding among these circadian studies is that RLS symptoms can be provoked at any time of day with sufficient imposed rest among patients with severe RLS.[8-10] This possibility can become important when evaluating RLS patients who develop augmentation (see *Chapter 9*). It may also have clinical relevance when the alleviation of nighttime symptoms leads to more attention to the afternoon RLS symptoms. In other words, even without the temporal advance to earlier onset of RLS symptoms due to augmentation, treated RLS patients may begin to feel that they need relief from RSL symptoms earlier in the day.

5. *Solely Not Accounted For by Other Medical or Behavioral Conditions*

There are two main categories of conditions that can be confused with RLS. First, there is the condition of restlessness, which can range from true akathisia to generalized anxiety. Indeed, the most severe or augmented RLS can resemble generalized akathisia

FIGURE 2.1 — Circadian Rhythm of RLS and Core Temperature

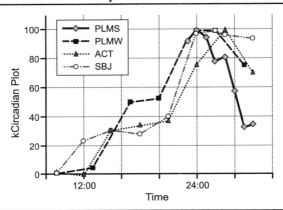

Key: ACT, activity accounts (measure of motor restlessness); mSIT, modified SIT to allow restless movement to alleviate symptoms; PLMS, periodic limb movements in sleep; PSG, polysomnography; PLMW, periodic limb movements while awake; SBJ, subjective leg discomfort; SIT, suggested immobilization test.

Circadian composite figure (reporting data from two studies[1,2]). Normalized values of the RLS measures are plotted against clock time from 8:00 through 24:00 to 8:00. Hours represent beginning of a SIT period or beginning of an hour of enumerating PLMS. Hourly averages from the first study from 23:00 to 7:00 are plotted as percent of the maximum (94.9 per hour in the period from 24:00 to 1:00). Mean value for eight subjects and two nights PSG. All these are plotted as percent from minimum (0%) to maximum (100%). PLMW[1]—minimum of 13.8/hour (9:00), maximum of 91.5/hour (2:00). ACT[2]—minimum of 124.9 counts (12:00), maximum of 447.8 (3:00). SBJ[2]—minimum of 2.96 (on 0 to 10 scale averaged over 5 determinations per 1 hour mSIT) at 9:00; maximum of 6.04 (at 12:00). The values of PLMW[1], ACT[2], and SBJ[2] were taken by averaging daytime SITs (or mSITs) from the first 2 days of study; values from hours between 11:00 and 6:00 were taken from the night of sleep deprivation.

[1] Trenkwalder C, et al. *Mov Disord.* 1999;14:102-110.

[2] Hening WA, et al. *Sleep.* 1999;22:901-912.

and the symptoms of anxiety are both common in RLS and partially overlap the key features of RLS.[12] The main overlap is in an urge to move or discomfort at rest. **Table 2.4** lists the disorders in this category. Second, there are those disorders that involve pain or unpleasant feelings in the legs. Leg cramps, known in the United States as "charley horses," are typical of this category. **Table 2.5** lists disorders in this category of leg discomfort.

TABLE 2.4 — Disorders of Restlessness

Akathisia
- Due to neuroleptic or other dopamine-blocking medications
- Due to other classes of psychoactive compounds, such as selective serotonin reuptake inhibitors (SSRIs)
- Due to degenerative disease
- Idiopathic

Anxiety Disorders

Other Psychiatric Disorders
- Mania
- Obsessive-compulsive disorder

Repetitive Movement Habits
- Leg shaking
- Foot tapping

Leg Symptoms With Toe Dyskinesias
- Painful legs and moving toes
- "Painless legs" and moving toes

Movement Disorders[1]
- Hypnic jerks
- Propriospinal myoclonus at sleep onset
- Tic disorder
- Hypnic myoclonus:
  - Excessive fragmentary myoclonus
- Rhythmic movement disorder:
  - Hypnic foot tremor
  - Alternating leg movement activity

[1] American Sleep Disorders Association. *The International Classification of Sleep Disorders: Diagnostic and Coding Manual*. 2nd version. Chicago, IL: American Association of Sleep Disorders; 2005.

TABLE 2.5 — Disorders of Leg Discomfort

Cramps
- Nocturnal leg cramps
- Metabolic cramps
- Myopathic cramps

Arthritic Conditions
- Rheumatoid arthritis
- Osteoarthritis

Pain Syndromes
- Fibromyalgia
- Somatiform pain disorder

Vascular Disorders
- Claudication
- Varicose veins
- Berger's disease
- Diabetic small-vessel disease

Nerve Disorders
- Polyneuropathies:
  – Small-fiber neuropathies
  – Diabetic neuropathy
- Radiculopathies

It should be noted, however, that RLS can be comorbid with several conditions that are in the differential diagnosis, such as rheumatoid arthritis,[13] diabetic neuropathy,[14] or other pain syndromes.[15] These situations in which symptoms overlap can present some of the most difficult diagnostic quandaries.

■ **How to Avoid Misdiagnosis**

The first step in the differential diagnosis of RLS is to probe for the presence of the first four diagnostic features. For a secure diagnosis, all four must be present. Many of the mimic conditions will fail one or more of the four diagnostic features, such as the presence of an experienced urge to move or the lack of any history of a nighttime accentuation. In addition, some mimics that might cause problems for an epidemiologic study, such as positional discomfort or occasional nocturnal leg cramps, are unlikely to present within a clinical practice.

The next step, in doubtful cases, is to probe more deeply into the nature of the four features; some helpful questions to ask are given in **Table 2.6**. Such questioning may be necessary because simply asking about the four diagnostic features may not fully establish the core elements of the features.

In addition, there are aspects of RLS symptoms that go beyond the four features. You can ask about specific ways in which the symptoms manifest. A list of potential questions with an explanation of how the answers influence diagnosis is presented in **Table 2.7**.

TABLE 2.6 — Additional Questions to Ask to Elucidate the Five Diagnostic Features of RLS

Urge to Move
- Do you experience this urge within your legs?
- Is the need to move overwhelming to the point that you cannot resist moving your legs?
- Will the urge to move increase if you are in a confined position?

Provocation by Rest
- Do you have symptoms both sitting and lying?
- How long do you need to be at rest before your leg symptoms begin?
- Do your symptoms only begin when your legs are in a specific posture?

Relief by Activity
- How quickly do you get some relief when you start moving?
- Do your leg symptoms ever occur when you are walking?
- Do your leg symptoms ever start when you are walking?
- If you have obtained relief with walking, do the symptoms ever return while you continue to walk?

Circadian Rhythm
- When are your symptoms worst?
- When are your symptoms least?
- Do you find that your symptoms are less in the morning?

Mimics
- Will simply changing leg position by itself once without continuing to move usually relieve these feelings?
- Are these feelings due to muscle cramps?

TABLE 2.7 — Questions to Differentiate RLS From Mimics

1. How long do your symptoms last until you have full relief (you no longer need to move to obtain relief)?
   Restless leg syndrome (RLS) symptoms usually last at least 10 minutes and often hours before full relief is obtained.
2. Are your symptoms relieved if you merely make a single change in the posture of your legs?
   RLS symptoms are only briefly or occasionally benefited by a postural shift; in general, one shift will not have more than a transitory effect on a state of rest.
3. Are your symptoms like a sharp pain?
   While RLS symptoms may be described as painful, they generally present as a diffuse pain or ache.
4. Does pressing the involved part of the leg cause additional pain?
   In RLS, there is normally not tenderness; instead, pressing or rubbing may relieve discomfort.

Finally, there are features of patient presentation in history or on exam that can be used to discriminate different mimic conditions from RLS. Some of these are presented in **Table 2.8**. In cases with atypical features, such as arm predominance or the lack of any symptoms when at rest, one of the supportive features may help clarify the diagnosis or at least direct further investigation.

■ **Restless Legs Syndrome and the Fifth Edition of *Diagnostic Statistical Manual of Mental Disorders* (DSM-5)**

Used in both clinical and research settings, *Diagnostic and Statistical Manual of Mental Disorders* (DSM) is the standard classification of mental disorders used by mental health professionals in the United States and contains a listing of diagnostic criteria for ever psychiatric disorder recognized by the US health care system. The current edition, DSM-IV-TR, is used by professionals in a wide array of contexts, including psychiatrists and other physicians, psychologists,

TABLE 2.8 — Specific Issues in Differential Diagnosis

Disorder	Key Point
Akathisia	Can usually identify the causative agent
Anxiety	Even if there is a circadian rhythm, specific symptoms in the legs are absent
Leg shaking/foot tapping	Usually do not experience an urge to move
Painful legs and moving toes	Exam discloses 1 to 2 Hz movements of the toes
Cramps	Usually intensely painful with obvious muscle contraction
Arthritis	Location of pain and signs to the joints
Pain syndromes	May have no urge to move and unusual distribution
Nerve disorders	Frequent numbness and signs of muscle wasting

social workers, nurses, occupational and rehabilitation therapists, and counselors, as well as by clinicians and researchers. In addition to supplying detailed descriptions of diagnostic criteria for each psychiatric disorder, DSM is also a necessary tool for communicating diagnosis of psychiatric disorders among clinicians who treat patients and academics who engage in research.

Previously, RLS was not listed in DSM-IV and was subsumed under the diagnostic category of Dyssomnia Not Otherwise Specified. However, for the fifth edition of DSM (DSM-5; scheduled to be released in May 2013), RLS is elevated to its own diagnostic criteria based on the following rationale:

- Significant prevalence of RLS in the general population
- Association of RLS with significant clinical and functional impairment
- Identified and replicated genetic markers for RLS

- Successful treatment response of RLS
- Evidence for a defined pathophysiologic basis of RLS.

The elevation of RLS to a full diagnostic entity in DSM-5 again affirms the public health significance of RLS and scientific progress by the RLS researchers. The members of IRLSSG have worked with the Sleep Disorders Workgroup of DSM-5 to create a diagnostic criteria for RLS that are similar to the 2011 Revised IRLSSG diagnostic criteria. The updated version of the DSM-5 RLS Criteria is presented in **Table 2.9**.

The DSM-5 RLS Criteria are similar to the Revised Criteria in emphasizing the necessity of ascertaining the first four features of the Revised Criteria and requiring the consideration for mimics an differential diagnosis with criterion E—"The occurrence of the above symptoms (Criteria A) are not solely accounted for by another medical or behavioral condition (eg, positional discomfort, leg cramps, habitual foot tapping, arthritis, leg edema, and peripheral ischemia)."

The difference between the two criteria lies in the handling of the "clinical significance." The Revised Criteria aimed to provide a broad diagnostic criteria for all forms and severity of RLS by not including "clinical significance" or frequency/ duration requirement in its diagnostic criteria. Instead, the Revised Criteria opts to specify more severe RLS that merits clinical attention by providing "a clinical significance specifier." Similarly, the Revised Criteria utilizes the course specifier to differentiate "chronic-persistent" form of RLS from the "intermittent" form. In contrast, DSM-5 RLS Criteria aimed to categorize clinically significant RLS only by requiring demonstration of clinical significance based on criterion B—"These symptoms are accompanied by significant distress or impairment in social, occupational, educational, academic, behavioral, or other important areas of functioning…" Frequency and duration requirements for DSM-5 Criteria for RLS remain undetermined as of May 1, 2012.[16]

TABLE 2.9 — Proposed Restless Legs Syndrome DSM-5 Criteria

A. Each of the following criteria must be met. The patient reports:

1. An urge to move the legs, usually accompanied or caused by uncomfortable and unpleasant sensations in the legs (for pediatric RLS, the description of these symptoms should be in the child's own words).

2. The symptoms begin or worsen during periods of rest or inactivity.

3. Symptoms are partially or totally relieved by movement.

4. Symptoms are worse in the evening or at night than during the day or occur only in the night/evening.

B. These symptoms are accompanied by significant distress or impairment in social, occupational, educational, academic, behavioral, or other important areas of functioning indicated by the presence of at least one of the following:

1. Clinical sleep disturbance (eg, significant sleep onset or maintenance problems, nocturnal awakenings, nonrestorative sleep)

2. Fatigue or low energy

3. Daytime sleepiness

4. Cognitive impairments (eg, attention, concentration, memory, learning)

5. Mood disturbance (eg, irritability, dysphoria, anxiety)

6. Behavioral problems (eg, hyperactivity, impulsivity, aggression)

7. Impaired academic, educational, or occupational function

8. Impaired interpersonal/social functioning

9. Negative impact on caregiver or family functioning (eg, fatigue, sleepiness)

C. Frequency: Remains under discussion

D. Duration: Remains under discussion

E. The occurrence of the above symptoms (Criteria A) are not solely accounted for by another medical or behavioral condition (eg, positional discomfort, leg cramps, habitual foot tapping, arthritis, leg edema, and peripheral ischemia).

F. The sleep difficulty occurs despite adequate age-appropriate circumstances and opportunity for sleep.

The 2002 IRLSSG-NIH consensus conference on RLS diagnosis indicated three specific findings that might enhance the likelihood of RLS diagnosis (**Table 2.10**); these include:

- The presence of PLM
- The response of symptoms to dopaminergics
- A positive family history.

TABLE 2.10 — Supportive Criteria for the Diagnosis of RLS

- The presence of an increased number or frequency of periodic limb movements for age
- The relief of symptoms by dopaminergic medications
- A family history of restless legs syndrome in close family members

Modified from Allen RP, et al. *Sleep Med.* 2003;4(2):101-119.

■ **Periodic Limb Movements**

These are common repetitive leg movements that are usually occur during sleep, but in RLS, they could occur while awake. The close association between PLM and RLS was first reported by the Lugaresi group in Bologna in the mid 1960s.[17,18] The diagnosis of PLM has been operationalized,[19] as reflected in the International Classification of Sleep Disorders-2[20] and the American Sleep Scoring Manual.[21] The criteria for PLM are given in **Table 2.11**. These movements occur in at least four or more (by definition) times, typically recur at intervals of 10 to 50 seconds (**Figure 2.2**), and can vary in period and amplitude with sleep/wake states.[22] As shown in the figure, the arms as well as the legs may be involved in the periodic limb movements in sleep (PLMS).[23] Most PLMS (see **Table 1.2** for definitions) occur during stages 1 and 2 non–rapid eye movement (NREM) sleep. Periodic increases and amplitude decreases in slower NREM sleep.[24] In REM sleep, amplitude and period may both

TABLE 2.11 — Current Diagnosis of Periodic Limb Movement

- Each movement (measured by EMG or actigraphy) lasts between 0.5 and 10 seconds
- The period of movements (interval from onset to onset) is at least 5 and not >90 seconds.
- For EMG, movement is said to begin when the rectified EMG rises 8 microvolts above baseline
- For EMG, movement is said to end when the rectified EMG falls below 2 microvolts above baseline for 0.5 seconds
- Movements must be separated by at least 0.5 seconds
- If a movement in one leg begins within 5 seconds of a movement in the other, it can be considered as part of the same movement
- At least four consecutive movements must meet the above criteria

Adapted from Zucconi M, et al. *Sleep Med.* 2006;7(2):175-183.

decrease. In wake, periodic limb movements in wake (PLMW) may be more irregular with a shorter period and a more prolonged duration of muscular activity that often includes muscular jerks.[25] These prolonged movements may include voluntary components evoked by the involuntary PLMW. A specific criterion of periodicity has been imposed to better define these movements: How regular are the successive intervals between movements?[26] In RLS, compared with other conditions, the PLMS are more regular, more strictly periodic. This is reflected in an index that forms a ratio between more periodic and less periodic movements.

Epidemiology of PLM

PLM are by no means restricted to those with RLS. In fact, it is more common to have PLM without RLS than have both PLM and RLS. Nevertheless, there seems to be an important pathophysiologic linkage between RLS as several genetic studies have reported association of PLMS with RLS in two reported genetic linkages, 12q[27] and 14q,[28,29] as well as one of the genes associated with RLS, BTB09 (6p).[29] One study

FIGURE 2.2 — Periodic Limb Movements in Sleep in a Patient With RLS

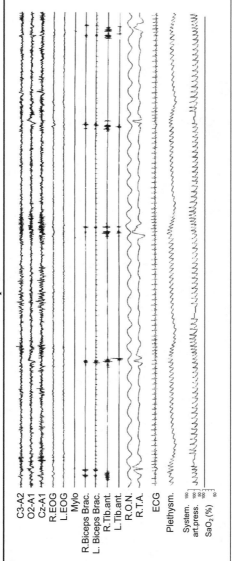

Key: Biceps Brac, biceps brachii; ECG, electrocardiogram; EOG, electrooculogram; L, left; Mylo, mylohyoideus; Plethysm, pletysmogram; PLMS, periodic limb movements during sleep; R, right; RON, oronasal respirogram; RTA, thoraco-abdominal respirogram; SaO$_2$, oxygen saturation; System art press, Systemic arterial pressure; Tib. ant, Tibialis anterior.

Contractions synchronously involve lower- and upper-limb muscles, recurring periodically about every 20 seconds. Note the ECG (heart rate) and plethysmogram (blood pressure) increases associated with the PLMS.

Courtesy of the Bologna Sleep Neurology group, Drs. Provini, Vertrugno, and Montagna.

also suggested that higher risk of PLMS among older individuals with RLS-suffering relatives than those without.[30] This finding is consistent with genetic determinants that are common to RLS and increased PLM.

Most studies of PLM have focused on those that occur during sleep or PLMS (see **Table 1.2** for definitions). The PLMS is frequent in the elderly.[31,32] Some studies in a general population indicate that PLMS are relatively infrequent (<5/hour of sleep) in during early decades of life, but frequency increases rapidly after age 40 and may continue to increase in older age groups (**Figure 2.3**).[33] In addition, PLMS in older subjects tend to be more rhythmic.

Table 2.12 lists conditions in which frequent PLMS have been found. Particularly noteworthy are such sleep neurologic conditions such as narcolepsy[34,35] and REM sleep behavior disorder,[36,37] two conditions that may also co-occur.[36]

FIGURE 2.3 — Distribution of Periodic Limb Movements During Sleep by Age

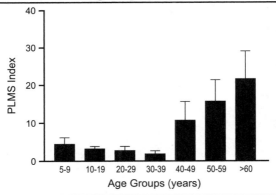

Mean PLMS index for healthy subjects according to 7 age groups (5-9 y, 10-19 y, 20-29 y, 30-39 y, 40-49 y, 50-59 y, and 60 y and older). Vertical bars represent the SEM.

Pennestri MH, et al. *Sleep*. 2006;29:1183-1187.

TABLE 2.12 — Conditions Other Than RLS With Frequent Periodic Limb Movement in Sleep

- Rapid eye movement behavior disorder
- Narcolepsy
- Synucleinopathies:
  - Parkinson's disease
  - Multiple-system atrophy
- Pregnancy (especially multiple pregnancies)
- Heart failure (post-transplant)
- Obstructive sleep apnea
- Antidepressant therapy:
  - Selective serotonin reuptake inhibitors
  - Tricyclic agents
  - Lithium

Association of PLM With RLS and Diagnostic Utility

The difficulty with using PLM as a diagnostic measure of RLS is that PLM are not specific for RLS. The Montreal group under Jacques Montplaisir has investigated the diagnostic utility of PLM for RLS. In an early study, the group found that 80% of RLS patients have >5 PLMS/hour sleep.[38] Subsequent studies used a combination of a SIT with a PSG sleep study to determine how well the combination of these two tests could differentiate between RLS patients and normal controls.[39] Using the measure of sensory discomfort—the subject's rating on a 10-point VAS—in the SIT combined with the index of PLMW (PLMW/hour of wake) during the PSG best differentiated the RLS subjects from controls with 82% sensitivity and 100% specificity. Therefore, the combination of high discomfort on the SIT and frequent PLMW at night is very uncommon in those who have few sleep complaints. On the other hand, the optimized measures they chose were not met by one of six RLS patients. The problem with this analysis is that it is unclear that when a more difficult differential diagnosis is required, say between RLS and polyneuropathy, a similarly effective discrimination can be made.

As discussed in *Chapter 3*, a PSG is not indicated for routine diagnosis of RLS. However, the detection of PLMS does require a PSG, and assessment of PLMS can be a reason for a PSG. Another available alternative diagnostic instrument is actigraphy. Small, accelerometer-based instruments that can be worn for several days and record and count PLM can be used to measure PLM.[40] Actigraphies are less expensive and allow for a longer recording than PSG does. This is useful since PLM may vary from day to day and can be better characterized with multiday recording.[41]

Periodic Limb Movement Disorder

An unresolved issue in sleep medicine is the clinical significance of PLMS.[42] Patients often have many PLMS without any sleep complaints, despite having PLMS associated with impair the quality of sleep.[43] Periodic limb movement disorder (PLMD) is a diagnosis in which PLMS are found to cause a specific complaint of disrupted sleep or excessive daytime sleepiness.[20] Specific diagnostic criteria are given in **Table 2.13**. To reach a diagnosis of PLMD, no other sleep-related diagnosis can account for the patient's complaint. Therefore, by definition, a patient with RLS cannot have PLMD. The diagnostic differences between RLS and PLMD are described in **Table 2.14**.

In general, leg movements, even if periodic, are not considered to be PLM if they are regularly associated with respiratory disturbances, such as sleep apnea.[20] A respiratory disturbance of increased pressure and turbulence, usually heard as snoring, is called upper airway resistance syndrome (UARS).[44] Diagnosis of UARS requires monitoring of nasal or esophageal pressure during PSG. Therefore, many cases of insomnia or daytime sleepiness thought due to PLMD may be attributable to UARS. A potential association between PLMS and autonomic activation, including increases in heart rate and blood pressure, has been noted. The effect is greater if the PLMS are associated with an arousal.[45] This could provide

TABLE 2.13 — Diagnostic Criteria for Periodic Limb Movement Disorder

- Polysomnography demonstrates repetitive, highly stereotyped limb movements that are:
  - 10 seconds in duration;
  - In a sequence of four or more movements
  - Separated by an interval of >5 seconds (from limb movement onset to limb movement onset) and <90 seconds (typically there is an interval of 20 seconds to 40 seconds)[a]
- The PLMS Index exceeds five per hour in children and 15 per hour in most adult cases.
- There is clinical sleep disturbance or complaints of daytime fatigue. If PLMS are present without clinical sleep disturbance, the PLMS can be noted as a polysomnographic finding, but criteria are not met for a diagnosis of PLMD.
- The periodic limb movements are not better explained by another current sleep disorder, medical/neurologic disorder, medication use, or substance use disorder. An example would be the occurrence of periodic leg movements at the termination of cyclically occurring apneas, which should not be counted as true PLMS or PLMD

[a] The ICSD2 criteria use an obsolete measure of amplitude, which is no longer accepted.

Adapted from American Sleep Disorders Association. *The International Classification of Sleep Disorders: Diagnostic and Coding Manual.* 2nd version. Chicago, IL: American Association of Sleep Disorders; 2005.

biological underpinning of RLS as a risk factor for the development of cardiovascular disease, a finding frequently reported associated with RLS.[46,47]

■ Response to Dopaminergic Medications

The benefit of dopaminergic medications in treating RLS were reported several decades ago. Beginning with Akpinar's original report in 1982,[48] the vast majority of RLS treatment studies with dopaminergic medications have been successful.[49,50] This led to the widely accepted notion that lack of treatment response

TABLE 2.14 — Differences Between RLS and Periodic Limb Movement Disorder

	RLS	PLMD
Diagnosis	Clinical history with exclusion of mimics	Documentation of PLMS of sufficient quantity by PSG (or possibly actigraphy)
Complaint	Typical leg symptoms satisfying clinical features	Complaint of sleep disturbance or daytime excessive somnolence
Differential diagnosis	A variety of disorders involving an urge to move and leg complaints	Movement disorders of sleep, such as nocturnal epilepsy, RBD, rhythmic movement disorder
Treatment	Dopaminergics, anticonvulsants, opioids, sedative-hypnotics	Mostly dopaminergics, sedative-hypnotics, some anticonvulsants

to dopaminergic medication in previously untreated RLS patient raises questions about the validity of RLS diagnosis. In one study, individuals with possible RLS, not fulfilling all criteria, were tested by administering a single 100-mg dose of levodopa when they were symptomatic.[51] They then completed a VAS scale for severity of their RLS-like symptoms in two areas (urge to move and leg discomfort). Those who showed a ≥50% benefit on the scale were subsequently found to have true RLS. The dopaminergic challenge reportedly identified 83% and 90% of those with true RLS based on the VAS rating in two domains. This study supports clinical impression that giving a single trial dose of levodopa in a doubtful RLS case may aid the diagnostic validity. Further study is needed to establish the clinical value.

■ **Presence of a Positive Family History**

As explained in *Chapter 4*, idiopathic RLS is a familial disease with likely a genetic basis. Because of this, someone with a first-degree family member with RLS is up to six times more likely to have RLS than those without. These individuals are likely to be more familiar with the condition and better understand the symptoms. There are no studies on how useful a known positive family history is in uncertain cases, but family history is an important element in diagnostic evaluation for a pediatric RLS (see *Chapter 3*).

2

REFERENCES

1. Walters AS. Toward a better definition of the restless legs syndrome. International Restless Legs Syndrome Study Group. *Mov Disord*. 1995;10:634-642.

2. Allen RP, Picchietti D, Hening WA, et al. Restless legs syndrome: diagnostic criteria, special considerations, and epidemiology. A report from the restless legs syndrome diagnosis and epidemiology workshop at the National Institutes of Health. *Sleep Med*. 2003;4:101-119.

3. HeningWA, Allen RP, Washburn M, Lesage SR, Earley CJ. The four diagnostic criteria for Restless Legs Syndrome are unable to exclude confounding conditions ("mimics"). *Sleep Med*. 2009;10(9):976-981.

4. Michaud M, Chabli A, Lavigne G, Montplaisir J. Arm restlessness in patients with restless legs syndrome. *Mov Disord*. 2000;15:289-293.

5. Bassetti CL, Mauerhofer D, Gugger M, Mathis J, Hess CW. Restless legs syndrome: a clinical study of 55 patients. *Eur Neurol*. 2001;45:67-74.

6. Hening WA, Allen RP, Washburn M, Lesage S, Earley CJ. Validation of the Hopkins telephone diagnostic interview for restless legs syndrome. *Sleep Med*. 2008;9(3):283-289.

7. Michaud M, Dumont M, Paquet J, Desautels A, Fantini ML, Montplaisir J. Circadian variation of the effects of immobility on symptoms of restless legs syndrome. *Sleep*. 2005;28:843-846.

8. Allen RP, Dean T, Earley CJ. Effects of rest-duration, time-of-day and their interaction on periodic leg movements while awake in restless legs syndrome. *Sleep Med*. 2005;6:429-434.

9. Trenkwalder C, Hening WA, Walters AS, Campbell SS, Rahman K, Chokroverty S. Circadian rhythm of periodic limb movements and sensory symptoms of restless legs syndrome. *Mov Disord*. 1999;14:102-110.

10. Hening WA, Walters AS, Wagner M, et al. Circadian rhythm of motor restlessness and sensory symptoms in the idiopathic restless legs syndrome. *Sleep*. 1999;22:901-912.

11. Michaud M, Dumont M, Selmaoui B, Paquet J, Fantini ML, Montplaisir J. Circadian rhythm of restless legs syndrome: relationship with biological markers. *Ann Neurol*. 2004;55:372-380.

12. Lee HB, Hening WA, Allen RP, et al. Restless legs syndrome is associated with DSM-IV major depressive disorder and panic disorder in the community. *J Neuropsychiatry Clin Neurosci.* 2008;20(1):101-105.

13. Salih AM, Gray RE, Mills KR, Webley M. A clinical, serological and neurophysiological study of restless legs syndrome in rheumatoid arthritis. *Br J Rheumatol.* 1994;33:60-63.

14. Gemignani F, Brindani F, Vitetta F, Marbini A, Calzetti S. Restless legs syndrome in diabetic neuropathy: a frequent manifestation of small fiber neuropathy. *J Peripher Nerv Syst.* 2007;12:50-53.

15. Aigner M, Prause W, Freidl M, et al. High prevalence of restless legs syndrome in somatoform pain disorder. *Eur Arch Psychiatry Clin Neurosci.* 2007;257(1):54-57.

16. American Psychiatric Association DSM-5 Development. M 10 Restless Legs Syndrome. DSM-5 Web site: http://www.dsm5 .org/ProposedRevisions/Pages/proposedrevision.spx?rid=403#. Accessed March 13, 2013.

17. Lugaresi E, Cirignotta F, Coccagna G, Montagna P. Nocturnal myoclonus and restless legs syndrome. *Adv Neurol.* 1986;43: 295-307.

18. Lugaresi E, Coccagna G, Berti-Ceroni G, Ambrosetto C. Restless legs syndrome and nocturnal myoclonus. In: Gastaut H, ed. *The Abnormalities of Sleep in Man.* Bologna, Italy: Aulo Gaggi Editore; 1968:285-294.

19. Zucconi M, Ferri R, Allen R, et al. The official World Association of Sleep Medicine (WASM) standards for recording and scoring periodic leg movements in sleep (PLMS) and wakefulness (PLMW) developed in collaboration with a task force from the International Restless Legs Syndrome Study Group (IRLSSG). *Sleep Med.* 2006;7:175-183.

20. American Academy of Sleep Medicine. *International Classification of Sleep Disorders: Diagnostic and Coding Manual, 2nd Version.* Chicago, IL: American Association of Sleep Medicine; 2005.

21. American Academy of Sleep Medicine. *The AASM Manual for the Scoring of Sleep and Associated Events: Rules, Terminology and Technical Specification.* Westchester, IL: American Association of Sleep Medicine; 2007.

22. Pollmacher T, Schulz H. Periodic leg movements (PLM): their relationship to sleep stages. *Sleep.* 1993;16:572-577.

23. Chabli A, Michaud M, Montplaisir J. Periodic arm movements in patients with the restless legs syndrome. *Eur Neurol.* 2000;44:133-138.

2

24. Nicolas A, Michaud M, Lavigne G, Montplaisir J. The influence of sex, age and sleep/wake state on characteristics of periodic leg movements in restless legs syndrome patients. *Clin Neurophysiol*. 1999;110:1168-1174.

25. Michaud M, Poirier G, Lavigne G, Montplaisir J. Restless Legs Syndrome: scoring criteria for leg movements recorded during the suggested immobilization test. *Sleep Med*. 2001;2:317-321.

26. Ferri R, Zucconi M, Manconi M, et al. Different periodicity and time structure of leg movements during sleep in narcolepsy/cataplexy and restless legs syndrome. *Sleep*. 2006;29:1587-1594.

27. Desautels A, Turecki G, Montplaisir J, Sequeira A, Verner A, Rouleau GA. Identification of a major susceptibility locus for restless legs syndrome on chromosome 12q. *Am J Hum Genet*. 2001;69:1266-1270.

28. Bonati MT, Ferini-Strambi L, Aridon P, Oldani A, Zucconi M, Casari G. Autosomal dominant restless legs syndrome maps on chromosome 14q. *Brain*. 2003;126:1485-1492.

29. Stefansson H, Rye DB, Hicks A, et al. A genetic risk factor for periodic limb movements in sleep. *N Engl J Med*. 2007;357(7):639-647.

30. Birinyi PV, Allen RP, Hening W, Washburn T, Lesage S, Earley CJ. Undiagnosed individuals with first-degree relatives with restless legs syndrome have increased periodic limb movements. *Sleep Med*. 2006;7:480-485.

31. Ancoli-Israel S, Kripke DF, Mason W, Messin S. Sleep apnea and nocturnal myoclonus in a senior population. *Sleep*. 1981;4:349-358.

32. Ancoli-Israel S, Kripke DF, Mason W, Kaplan OJ. Sleep apnea and periodic movements in an aging sample. *J Gerontol*. 1985;40:419-425.

33. Pennestri MH, Whittom S, Adam B, Petit D, Carrier J, Montplaisir J. PLMS and PLMW in healthy subjects as a function of age: prevalence and interval distribution. *Sleep*. 2006;29:1183-1187.

34. Schenck CH, Mahowald MW. Motor dyscontrol in narcolepsy: rapid-eye-movement (REM) sleep without atonia and REM sleep behavior disorder. *Ann Neurol*. 1992;32:3-10.

35. Bahammam A. Periodic leg movements in narcolepsy patients: impact on sleep architecture. *Acta Neurol Scand*. 2007;115:351-355.

36. Schenck CH, Mahowald MW. Polysomnographic, neurologic, psychiatric, and clinical outcome report on 70 consecutive

cases with REM sleep behavior disorder (RBD): sustained clonazepam efficacy in 89.5% of 57 cases. *Cleve Clin J Med*. 1990;57(suppl):S9-S23.

37. Fantini ML, Michaud M, Gosselin N, Lavigne G, Montplaisir J. Periodic leg movements in REM sleep behavior disorder and related autonomic and EEG activation. *Neurology*. 2002;59: 1889-1894.

38. Montplaisir J, Boucher S, Poirier G, Lavigne G, Lapierre O, Lesperance P. Clinical, polysomnographic, and genetic characteristics of restless legs syndrome: a study of 133 patients diagnosed with new standard criteria. *Mov Disord*. 1997;12:61-65.

39. Michaud M, Paquet J, Lavigne G, Desautels A, Montplaisir J. Sleep laboratory diagnosis of restless legs syndrome. *Eur Neurol*. 2002;48:108-113.

40. Sforza E, Johannes M, Claudio B. The PAM-RL ambulatory device for detection of periodic leg movements: a validation study. *Sleep Med*. 2005;6:407-413.

41. Sforza E, Haba-Rubio J. Night-to-night variability in periodic leg movements in patients with restless legs syndrome. *Sleep Med*. 2005;6:259-267.

42. Mendelson WB. Are periodic leg movements associated with clinical sleep disturbance? *Sleep*. 1996;19:219-223.

43. Carskadon MA, Brown ED, Dement WC. Sleep fragmentation in the elderly: relationship to daytime sleep tendency. *Neurobiol Aging*. 1982;3:321-327.

44. Guilleminault C, Kim YD, Palombini L, Li K, Powell N. Upper airway resistance syndrome and its treatment. *Sleep*. 2000;23(suppl 4):S197-S200.

45. Pennestri MH, Montplaisir J, Colombo R, Lavigne G, Lanfranchi PA. Nocturnal blood pressure changes in patients with restless legs syndrome. *Neurology*. 2007;68:1213-1218.

46. Winkelman JW, Finn L, Young T. Prevalence and correlates of restless legs syndrome symptoms in the Wisconsin Sleep Cohort. *Sleep Med*. 2006;7:545-552.

47. Walters AS, Rye DB. Review of the relationship of restless legs syndrome and periodic limb movements in sleep to hypertension, heart disease, and stroke. *Sleep*. 2009;32(5):589-597.

48. Akpinar S. Treatment of restless legs syndrome with levodopa plus benserazide. *Arch Neurol*. 1982;39:739.

49. Littner MR, Kushida C, Anderson WM, et al. Practice parameters for the dopaminergic treatment of restless legs syndrome and periodic limb movement disorder. *Sleep*. 2004;27:557-559.

50. Vignatelli L, Billiard M, Clarenbach P, et al. EFNS guidelines on management of restless legs syndrome and periodic limb movement disorder in sleep. *Eur J Neurol*. 2006;13:1049-1065.

51. Stiasny-Kolster K, Kohnen R, Moller JC, Trenkwalder C, Oertel WH. Validation of the "L-DOPA test" for diagnosis of restless legs syndrome. *Mov Disord*. 2006;21:1333-1339.

3

Who Gets RLS and How Does It Progress?

Epidemiology of RLS

RLS is a common disorder in Western populations. According to a recent systematic review, reported general prevalence rates of RLS in North American and Western European populations ranges from 4% to 29% of adults, averaging 14.5%+/- 8.0% across studies.[1] The wide variation in prevalence estimates is likely due to inconsistencies in RLS diagnostic criteria and procedures among the studies. Prevalence of RLS decreases as defining criteria increase in strictness in European and North American general adult population. When a set of three or four symptoms meeting minimal diagnostic criteria of the 2002 NIH/IRLSSG Consensus meeting is applied, prevalence estimates ranges from 3.9% to 14.3%.

However, the 2011 revised diagnostic criteria for RLS recommends adding the fifth criterion that emphasizes importance of evaluation for "mimics" and consideration for differential diagnoses before making a firm diagnosis of RLS (see *Chapter 2*). When differential diagnosis is applied, prevalence estimates have been reported to range from 1.9% to 4.6%.[2] Prevalence of clinically significant RLS—defined as frequency of more than twice a week with at least moderate distress—has been estimated to be 2.7% according to the REST general population study that examined 16,202 participants in five European countries and United States.[3]

Studies of other populations have resulted in highly variable results. Some Asian studies have found a very low prevalence of RLS in the general population (<1%),[4,5] others have found an intermediate level (1%

to 4%),[6,7] while still others have found a prevalence to be near the Western population range (5% to 10%).[8,9] Interestingly, even when the RLS case ascertainment method and sampling strategies are similar, prevalence of RLS seems to be substantially lower among Asians in comparison with the Western populations (**Figure 3.1**). Differences in culture and risk factors that affect the expression of RLS appear to vary between Asian and Western countries.

There are other reports of ethnic variability as well, but data are scant. For example, one study in South American Indian populations found an intermediate prevalence, higher at altitude.[10] However, because of variability in case ascertainment methods and sampling strategies, it is difficult as of yet to make a clear determination of the prevalence estimates. This point is

FIGURE 3.1 — RLS Prevalence Figures by Gender in the Primary Care REST Study

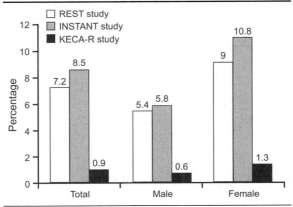

This figure demonstrates variability of prevalence estimates across the three studies that utilized similar sampling frames and RLS case ascertainment methods. The KECA-R study conducted in South Korea shows prevalence of RLS substantially lower than the REST study and INSTANT study conducted in Western Countries.

Cho SJ, et al. *Sleep*. 2009;32(8):1069-1076.

underlined by a population-based study that found no RLS prevalence disparity between African Americans and whites in the same community, although African American RLS patients are uncommon in specialty clinics.[11]

■ Risk Factors

Table 3.1 summarizes risk factors for RLS identified from different studies. The most important general population risk factors are age and sex.

TABLE 3.1 — Risk Factors for Development of RLS

Demographic Factors
- Older age[a]
- Female sex[a]
- Living at higher altitude
- Lower socioeconomic status

Lifestyle Factors
- Lack of exercise
- Smoking

Medical Conditions
General
- Pregnancy[a]
- Poor physical health
- Poor mental health
- Obesity

Specific Disorders
- Iron deficiency and anemia[a]
- Renal failure[a]
- Polyneuropathy
- Diabetes
- Parkinson's disease
- Multiple sclerosis
- Hypothyroidism
- Gastric resection
- B_{12} deficiency
- Spinocerebellar ataxia type 3: Machado-Joseph disease
- Lung transplant
- Magnesium deficiency

[a] These are best established risk factors.

Age

The risk of RLS rises with age. Most studies have looked only at adults, but a population study of children indicates that prevalence also rises during the childhood years, with 0.5% of children 8 to 12 and 1.0% of children 13 to 17 having RLS.[12] Some studies have shown that beyond age 65 or 70, there may be a decrease in incidence of RLS. The explanation for this decline is unknown and may relate either to biologic factors or to response factors (the oldest individuals may be less likely to endorse RLS symptoms).

Sex

Women have about twice the risk of developing RLS as men. The figures from some studies are given in **Table 3.2**. Two studies have found that RLS is increased in women who have been pregnant; the frequency of RLS in never-pregnant women was not significantly different from that of men.[13,14] In the German study, frequency of RLS also increased with additional pregnancies, so that the risk for women with three or more pregnancies was 3.57 that of men.[13] Pregnancy is also an immediate cause for RLS: between 20% and 25% of pregnant women have RLS, with more than half of them developing the condition for the first time during pregnancy.

Family History

RLS has a familial component in many cases. Several epidemiologic studies have examined and confirmed a family history of RLS. Up to 60% of individuals with RLS have a positive family history. As discussed later, those who are related to RLS patients are more likely to have RLS.[15,16] A twin study has reported a high RLS concordance rate (83.3%) between identical twins, but the same study reported variability in age of onset, disease severity, and symptom descriptions and suggested environmental contribution to development and progression of RLS in familial cases.[17] While familial and non-familial RLS share

TABLE 3.2 — RLS Symptom Prevalence in Men and Women

Study Author	Location	Overall (%)	Men (%)	Women (%)
Ulfberg 2001[a,1,2]	Sweden	—	5.8	11.4
Sevim 2003[3]	Turkey	3.2	2.5	3.9
Berger 2004[4]	Germany	10.4	7.6	13.4
Allen 2005[5]	Europe-USA	7.2	5.4	9.0
Bjorvatn 2005[6]	Scandinavia	11.5	9.4	13.4
Hogl 2005[7]	Italian Tirol	10.6	6.6	14.2
Cho 2008[8]	Korea	6.2	8.7	7.5
Tison 2005[9]	France	8.5	5.8	10.8

[a] Ulfberg did separate studies for men and women.

[1] Ulfberg J, et al. *Eur Neurol.* 2001;46:17-19.

[2] Ulfberg J, et al. *Mov Disord.* 2001;16:1159-1163.

[3] Sevim S, et al. *Neurology.* 2003;61:1562-1569.

[4] Berger K, et al. *Arch Intern Med.* 2004;164:196-202.

[5] Allen RP, et al. *Arch Intern Med.* 2005;165:1286-1292.

[6] Bjorvatn B, et al. *Sleep Med.* 2005;6:307-312.

[7] Hogl B, et al. *Neurology.* 2005;64:1920-1924.

[8] Cho YW, et al. *Sleep.* 2008;31:219-223.

[9] Tison F, et al. *Neurology.* 2005;65:239-246.

similar signs, symptoms, and clinical courses, familial RLS tends to be associated with earlier age of onset and more frequent worsening during pregnancy.[18]

Medical Conditions and Cardiovascular Risks

The most important and well-established conditions are iron deficiency and renal failure. Also, various studies have found that obesity (increased body mass index [BMI]), general poor health, and smoking may be related to an increased frequency of RLS symptoms. There is an emerging body of literature suggesting association between RLS and various cardiovascular risks such as diabetes, hypertension, obesity, and dyslipidemia.[19,20] Underlying mechanisms and direction of causality, however, remains unclear.

Mental Health and Psychiatric Medications

Depression and anxiety seem to be strongly associated with RLS. Many antidepressant medications and dopamine receptor–blocking agents, including both typical and atypical antipsychotic medications, may provoke RLS or aggravate preexisting symptoms. A more detailed discussion follows in *Chapter 12*.

■ Secondary RLS

The most important conditions that cause RLS are iron deficiency, renal failure, pregnancy, rheumatoid conditions, neuropathy, and diabetes. RLS may also be more common in patients with Parkinson's disease.

Iron Deficiency and Anemia

The finding that iron deficiency can cause RLS goes back to Ekbom; iron therapy was an early treatment studied.[21] In more recent years, this association has been confirmed.[22-24] Iron treatment, either oral or intravenous, may benefit RLS. As discussed in *Chapter 4*, a deficiency of brain iron may be a key mechanism of development for RLS. Bleeding conditions due to various causes (eg, nonsteroidal anti-inflammatory medications or cancer) can present with RLS.[25-28] Some studies have reported regular blood donation as a potential risk factor for RLS, but more recent studies have found conflicting results.[29-31]

Renal Failure

Studies have generally found an elevated frequency of RLS in renal patients,[32,33] although this has ranged from a low of 6.6% in India[5] to a high of 70% in Hong Kong, China.[34] There have been no consistent findings of specific factors that predispose to RLS, although this is a population that is, in general, both iron deficient and anemic. More aggressive modern treatment of anemia and iron deficiency with epoetin and intravenous iron may be reducing the frequency, but this has not been well demonstrated.

Pregnancy

Some 20% to 25% of women will have RLS during pregnancy.[35,36] More than half of these women develop RLS for the first time during pregnancy; in most of these with newly developed RLS, symptoms will remit near the time of delivery.

Rheumatoid Conditions

Patients with select rheumatoid conditions, including rheumatoid arthritis,[37] scleroderma,[38] Sjogren's syndrome,[39] and fibromyalgia,[40] may experience increased RLS.

Neuropathy

It has long been suggested that RLS is associated with neuropathy, but one study found only a 5% frequency of RLS in neuropathy patients.[41] Two more studies from one group found a clearly increased frequency of RLS in both polyneuropathy[42] and diabetic neuropathy[43] patients.

Diabetes

Most epidemiologic studies have suggested that RLS is more common in diabetes. A case series study and a case-control study found that RLS is more frequent in diabetics, perhaps due to the associated neuropathy.[44,45]

Relationship to Parkinson's Disease

Parkinson's disease (PD) bears an unusual relationship to RLS. On the one hand, the same dopaminergic medications help both conditions. In other ways, they are quite different: Patients with PD have increased iron in the brain; those with RLS, low; PD affects more men; RLS, more women. Some studies have found an increased frequency of RLS,[46] but noted that most RLS began after PD, atypical for familial or idiopathic RLS.

Other Conditions

Other conditions that might cause RLS, some of which are only suggested, are presented in **Table 3**.1.

Genetics of RLS

■ Familial Aggregation

Several case series clearly established that more than half of RLS patients are aware of affected relatives.[47-49] This has since been confirmed by formal interview studies that diagnosed relatives directly,[50] clearly showing that patients with idiopathic RLS are more likely to have affected relatives than those with secondary RLS (due to renal failure). A best estimate of the increased risk to first-degree relatives of RLS patients is that they are about five times as likely to have RLS as are nonrelatives.[51] These studies do indicate that RLS runs in families, but this may be due either to genetics or to a shared common environment.

■ Segregation Analyses

One way to sort out genetic and environmental causes is to do a segregation analysis that determines the genetic model that best explains how a disorder runs in a family. At least, two previous have shown that the pattern of RLS in a family might be of a dominant inheritance (one abnormal allele determines disease likelihood) in some RLS families.[52,53] This supports the likelihood that some of the familial aggregation in

RLS is genetic. One of the studies also showed that the age at onset may be under genetic control.[53]

■ Linkage and Association Analyses

Direct genetic studies of RLS identified five suspect locations on six different chromosomes (**Table 3.3**). Near one of these, on 12q, an association has been found to the neuronal nitrogen oxide synthetase gene (NOS1).[54] Recently, three groups have reported associations linked to several specific genes, one confirmed in two studies (2p, 6p, 15q) (**Table 3.3**).[55-58] It is clear that RLS is a complex disorder and that there are a number of genetic and environmental factors that contribute to its causation.

The Clinical Picture of RLS

■ The Spectrum of Severity

RLS has a wide variety of severities from rare, non-disturbing episodes that are barely remembered to severe, almost unremitting, symptoms that last for most of the day and prevent most of sleep at night. In the community, several studies have suggested that:

- About 15% to 20% have daily or almost daily symptoms
- About 40% have at least weekly, but not daily symptoms
- About 40% have less than weekly symptoms.

The REST studies found that about one third of those identified as having RLS symptoms had symptoms sufficiently severe to merit medical intervention (defined as "bothersome symptoms that occur at least twice a week") in the general population[3] and in the primary care clinics.[57] More recent studies have confirmed using physician diagnosis that this group makes up 1% to 2% of the adult population. A study based on a German primary care sample reported that approximately a quarter of those with RLS are aware that they have RLS and that only every fifth patient with RLS desires medication to reduce their symptoms.[60]

TABLE 3.3 — Genetic Linkages and Associations in RLS

Linkages

Author	Population	Linkage	Model
RLS1—Desautels 2001[1]	French Canadian	12q	Recessive
RLS2—Bonafi 2003[2]	Italian	14q	Dominant
RLS3—Chen 2004[3]	United States	9p	Dominant
RLS4—Pichler 2006[4]	Italian Tirol	2q	Dominant
RLS5—Levchenko 2006[5]	French Canadian	20p	Dominant
RLS6—Levchenko 2009[6]	French Canadian	16p	Dominant

Associations

Author	Population	Chromosome	Gene
Winkelmann et al[7]	French Canadian/European	2p	MEIS1, exon 9
		6p	BTBD9, intron 5
		15q	MAP2K5, LBXCOR1
Stefannson et al[a,8]	Icelandic/United States	6p	BTBD9, intron
Schomair et al[9]	German	9p	PTPRD
Winkelmann et al[10]	European	12q	NOS1

62

[a] This association appears to be more related to increased periodic limb movements than to the subjective symptoms of RLS, but the Winkelmann association in the same gene was ascertained in a population defined by subjective symptoms.

[1] Desautels A, et al. *Am J Hum Genet.* 2001;69:1266-1270.

[2] Bonati MT, et al. *Brain.* 2003;126:1485-1492.

[3] Chen S, et al. *Am J Hum Genet.* 2004;74:876-885.

[4] Pichler I, et al. *Am J Hum Genet.* 2006;79:716-723.

[5] Levchenko A, et al. *Neurology.* 2006;67:900-901.

[6] Levchenko A, et al. *Mov Disord.* 2009;24:40-50.

[7] Winkelmann J, et al. *Nature Genet.* 2007;39(8):1000-1006.

[8] Stefansson H, et al. *N Engl J Med.* 2007;357:639-647.

[9] Schormair B, et al. *Nat Genet.* 2008;40:946-948.

[10] Winkelmann J, et al. *Mov Disord.* 2008;23:350-358.

3

Patients with mild RLS often have symptoms only when they are forced to spend long periods under restrained rest. As RLS worsens, it becomes more frequent and symptoms may be present for longer periods of the day. This is the basis of the Johns Hopkins RLS Severity Scale[61] (**Table 3.4**). In the patients with the most severe RLS, symptoms can be present for most of the day and may only be partially relieved with activity. In extreme cases, RLS crisis or "status" can occur.[62]

TABLE 3.4 — The Johns Hopkins RLS Severity Scale

Occurrence of RLS	Rating
No RLS	0
Less than daily RLS	0.5
RLS only beginning at bedtime or in the night	1
RLS beginning after 6 PM but before bedtime	2
RLS beginning before 6 PM	3
RLS beginning before noon	4

■ **The Course of RLS: RLS Is a Chronic Disorder**

RLS is usually a chronic condition for clinically significant RLS but can have variable courses for the mild type. In the Hopkins family study, >95% of those who had been diagnosed with clinically significant, idiopathic RLS continued to have it at the time of interview, for an average duration of almost 20 years. In contrast, family members, often with milder RLS symptoms, report that their course of RLS is stable, relapsing, or even improving over the years. Also, RLS patients usually describe a progressive course. Those with younger-age onset, most likely to be familial and idiopathic, describe a slowly progressive course of their condition. Those with later onset, often secondary, experience a more rapidly progressive course.[63]

It is important for a clinician to recognize the chronic nature of clinically significant RLS; it is not a disorder that can be treated acutely and cured, but must be managed over a span of many years like diabetes, hypertension, and cardiovascular disease.

RLS in Special Populations

There are additional considerations for diagnosing and managing RLS in special populations. Children can have distinctive features and require more circumspect dosing. Cognitively impaired adults may not be able to describe the key diagnostic features that are necessary to confirm the diagnosis. The phenomenology of RLS manifested in secondary RLS conditions also may vary from the typical picture of idiopathic RLS.

■ RLS in Children

Most adolescents, children ≥12 years of age, are capable of providing a clinical history sufficient to use the adult criteria for diagnosing RLS. However, children <12 years of age may not be able to describe their leg sensations or may give them juvenile terms (such as "owies" or "thingies"); they may be less aware of a circadian factor and most bothered in school, where they may be thought to have attention deficit hyperactivity disorder (ADHD).[64] This led to the 2002 NIH workshop to propose a more rigorous diagnostic scheme for children than for adults,[65] but which also utilized the supportive criteria of PLMS and family history (**Table 3.5**). In addition, particularly for research purposes, the workshop proposed that diagnosis of probable or possible RLS be considered for children who could not meet full diagnostic criteria (**Table 3.6**).

The 2011 Revised IRLSSG Diagnostic Criteria (**Table 2.1**) addresses diagnosis of RLS in children as well. An important caveat in diagnosis of RLS in children according to the Revised Criteria is the fact that consideration for differential diagnosis should include other pediatric conditions during the evaluation. Previous research has made it clear that children with RLS may have been mistakenly diagnosed with either ADHD[66,67] or growing pains.[68,69] Also, clinical

TABLE 3.5 — Diagnosis of RLS in Children (Under Approximately Age 12 Years)

Criteria for the Diagnosis of Definite RLS in Children

Child meets all four of the following adult criteria:
1. An urge to move the legs
2. The urge to move begins or worsens when sitting or lying down
3. The urge to move is partially or totally relieved by movement
4. The urge to move is worse in the evening or night than during the day or only occurs in the evening or night

and

The child uses his or her own words to describe leg discomfort. Examples of age-appropriate descriptors: owies, tickle, tingle, static, bugs, spiders, ants, boo-boos, want to run, and a lot of energy in my legs.

OR

Child meets all four of the above adult criteria and two or three of the following supportive criteria:
1. Sleep disturbance for age
2. Biological parent or sibling has definite RLS
3. The child has a sleep study documenting a periodic limb movement index of five or more per hour of sleep

Allen RP, et al. *Sleep Med.* 2003;4:101-119.

course of RLS in children remains unclear and the specifics for clinical course of RLS are difficult to be applied in children.

■ **RLS in the Cognitively Impaired Elderly**

RLS is primarily a clinical diagnosis based on careful ascertainment of key diagnostic features based on subjective report by the patient. Cognitively impaired, elderly patients often are not reliable in their report of symptoms due to deficits in various aspects of cognition and language, and an adequate assessment of these patients may not be possible. The 2002 NIH workshop offered some suggestions for how to

TABLE 3.6 — Research Diagnosis for Probable or Possible RLS in Children

Criteria for the Diagnosis of Probable RLS in Children

Child meets all four of the following adult criteria except #4:
1. An urge to move the legs
2. The urge to move begins or worsens when sitting or lying down
3. The urge to move is partially or totally relieved by movement
4. The urge to move is worse in the evening or night than during the day or only occurs in the evening or night

and

The child has a biological parent or sibling with definite RLS.

OR

The child is observed to have behavior manifestations of lower-extremity discomfort when sitting or lying, with motor movement of the affected limbs. The discomfort has characteristics of adult criteria 2, 3, and 4 above; worse during rest and inactivity, relieved by movement, and worse during the evening and night.

and

The child has a biological parent or sibling with definite RLS.

Criteria for the Diagnosis of Possible RLS in Children

The child has periodic limb movement disorder.

and

The child has a biologic parent or sibling with definite RLS, but the child does not meet definite or probable childhood RLS definitions.

Allen RP, et al. *Sleep Med.* 2003;4:101-119.

diagnose these individuals (**Table 3.7**). However, in patients with dementia, sundowning and diurnal pattern of behavioral disturbance is common, and their restless wandering is often difficult to distinguish from walking activities to relieve urge to move.

TABLE 3.7 — Diagnosis of RLS in Cognitively Impaired Elderly[a]

Historical Issues

- History of RLS diagnosed by a medical professional
- Family member's report of typical RLS features
- Affected family members
- Past evidence of a high number of PLMS
- Written evidence in which patient expresses RLS features

Current Observations

- Signs of leg discomfort, such as expressions of pain or attempts to rub, massage, or strike legs
- Excessive motor activity in legs, including fidgeting, shaking, pushing back and forth, twisting, flexing, and extending
- Signs of agitation and inability to stay still, excessive walking
- Inability to get to sleep because of restless activity and exaggerated motor activity during sleep period
- Resistance to restraint or increased signs of discomfort when seated
- Reduced indication of leg discomfort when active, moving, or walking
- Nocturnal accentuation of behavioral signs
- Observed or documents excessive PLM (>25/hour)

Review activity regulations and current medications to determine if RLS-provocative procedures or substances are present

[a] May be also applied to younger individuals who have cognitive limitations due to developmental issues, disease, or trauma.

Modified from Allen RP, et al. *Sleep Med.* 2003;4:101-119.

Also, a problem of RLS in this group, especially within secured or locked units such as nursing homes and rehabilitation centers, is that their behaviors might be subjected to a variety of factors that can induce or aggravate RLS, including restraint and psychoactive medications (eg, dopamine blockers and SSRI/SNRIs) that might provoke RLS symptoms. Therefore, the treating physician should consider RLS when sufficient features are present to warrant such diagnosis.

Minimizing the use of dopamine-blocking tranquilizers or SSRI/SNRIs for mood and other behavioral symptoms in those with RLS-like features should be attempted. Targeted treatment for RLS symptoms in this population should be started cautiously to avoid possible serious drug interactions since polypharmacy is often detrimental in this population.

■ RLS in Those with Secondary Disorders

As a general matter, the diagnosis of secondary RLS or RLS due to secondary medical conditions (eg, iron deficiency) usually proceeds in the same way as that of idiopathic RLS. However, the nature of the relationship—whether the co-occurring condition is a cause or comorbidity—needs to be carefully investigated. A thorough review on the time of onset of RLS symptoms and the secondary disorder and the temporal relationship between improvement and aggravation of the two conditions are factors that may help determine their relationship. For example, iron-deficiency anemia is common among women and elderly population, and the temporal relationship between RLS and iron-deficiency anemia is often difficult to establish. With or without RLS, iron deficiency anemia should be treated and treating and reversing a potentially etiologic cause of RLS with iron supplement would likely ameliorate the RLS symptoms as well. However, it is often the case that "bridge" or even permanent treatment with RLS-specific medications may be needed to manage the RLS symptoms.

REFERENCES

1. Innes KE, Selfe TK, Agarwal P. Prevalence of restless legs syndrome in North Aemrican and Western European populations: a systematic review. *Sleep Med*. 2012;12:623-634.

2. Ohayon MM, O'Hara R, Vitiello MV. Epidemiology of restless legs syndrome: a synthesis of the literature. *Sleep Med Rev*. 2012;16:283-295.

3. Allen RP, Walters AS, Montplaisir J, et al. Restless legs syndrome prevalence and impact: REST general population study. *Arch Intern Med*. 2005;165:1286-1292.

4. Tan EK, Seah A, See SJ, Lim E, Wong MC, Koh KK. Restless legs syndrome in an Asian population: a study in Singapore. *Mov Disord*. 2001;16:577-579.

5. Cho SJ, Hong JP, Hahm BJ, et al. Restless legs syndrome in a community sample of Korean adults: prevalence, impact on quality of life, and association with DSM-IV psychiatric disorders. *Sleep*. 2009;32(8):1069-1076.

6. Sevim S, Dogu O, Camdeviren H, et al. Unexpectedly low prevalence and unusual characteristics of RLS in Mersin, Turkey. *Neurology*. 2003;61:1562-1569.

7. Mizuno S, Miyaoka T, Inagaki T, Horiguchi J. Prevalence of restless legs syndrome in non-institutionalized Japanese elderly. *Psychiatry Clin Neurosci*. 2005;59:461-465.

8. Cho YW, Shin WC, Yun CH, et al. Epidemiology of restless legs syndrome in Korean adults. *Sleep*. 2008;31:219-223.

9. Rangarajan S, D'Souza GA. Restless legs syndrome in Indian patients having iron deficiency anemia in a tertiary care hospital. *Sleep Med*. 2007;8:247-251.

10. Castillo PR, Kaplan J, Lin SC, Fredrickson PA, Mahowald MW. Prevalence of restless legs syndrome among native South Americans residing in coastal and mountainous areas. *Mayo Clin Proc*. 2006;81:1345-1347.

11. Lee HB, Hening WA, Allen RP, Earley CJ, Eaton WW, Lyketsos CG. Race and restless legs syndrome symptoms in an adult community sample in east Baltimore. *Sleep Med*. 2006;7:642-645.

12. Picchietti D, Allen RP, Walters AS, Davidson JE, Myers A, Ferini Strambi I. Restless legs syndrome: prevalence and impact in children and adolescents, the Peds REST study. *Pediatrics*. 2007;120(2):253-266.

13. Berger K, Luedemann J, Trenkwalder C, John U, Kessler C. Sex and the risk of restless legs syndrome in the general population. *Arch Intern Med*. 2004;164:196-202.

14. Hening WA, Allen RP, Lasage S, Earley CJ. The risk of RLS depends on gender and history of pregnancy in a case-control family study. *Neurology*. 2007;68:A345. Abstract.

15. Tison F, Crochard A, Leger D, Bouee S, Lainey E, El Hasnaoui A. Epidemiology of restless legs syndrome in French adults: a nationwide survey: the INSTANT study. *Neurology*. 2005;65:239-246.

16. Vogl FD, Pichler I, Adel S, et al. Restless legs syndrome: epidemiological and clinicogenetic study in a South Tyrolean population isolate. *Mov Disord*. 2006;21:1189-1196.

17. Ondo WG, Vuong KD, Wang Q. Restless legs syndrome in monozygotic twins: clinical correlates. *Neurology*. 2000;55:1404-1406.

18. Winkelmann J, Wetter TC, Collado-Seidel, et al. Clinical characteristics and frequency of the hereditary restless legs syndrome in a population of 300 patients. *Sleep*. 2000;23:597-602.

19. Innes KE, Selfe TK, Agarwal P. Restless legs syndrome and conditions associated with metabolic dysregulation, sympathoadrenal dysfunction, and cardiovascular disease risk: a systematic review. *Sleep Med Rev*. 2012:16(4):309-339.

20. Walters AS, Rye DB. Review of the relationship of restless legs syndrome and periodic limb movements in sleep to hypertension, heart disease, and stroke. *Sleep*. 2009;32:589-597.

21. Nordlander NB. Therapy in restless legs. *Acta Med Scand*. 1953;145:453-457.

22. O'Keeffe ST, Noel J, Lavan JN. Restless legs syndrome in the elderly. *Postgrad Med J*. 1993;69:701-703.

23. O'Keeffe ST, Gavin K, Lavan JN. Iron status and restless legs syndrome in the elderly. *Age Ageing*. 1994;23:200-203.

24. Sun ER, Chen CA, Ho G, Earley CJ, Allen RP. Iron and the restless legs syndrome. *Sleep*. 1998;21:371-377.

25. Leutgeb U, Martus P. Regular intake of non-opioid analgesics is associated with an increased risk of restless legs syndrome in patients maintained on antidepressants. *Eur J Med Res*. 2002;7:368-378.

26. Ekbom KA. Restless legs as an early symptom of cancer. *Sven Lakartidn*. 1955;52:1875-1883.

27. Brocklehurst J. Restless legs syndrome as a presenting symptom in malignant disease. *Age Ageing*. 2003;32:234.

28. Morcos Z. Restless legs syndrome, iron deficiency and colon cancer. *J Clin Sleep Med*. 2005;1:433.

29. Silber MH, Richardson JW. Multiple blood donations associated with iron deficiency inpatients with restless legs syndrome. *Mayo Clin Proc*. 2003;78:52-54.

30. Arunthari V, Kaplan J, Frederickson PA, Lin SC, Castillo PR, Heckman MS. Prevalence of restless legs syndrome in blood donors. *Mov Disord*. 2010;25;1451-1455.

31. Burchell BJ, Allen RP, Miller JK, Hening WA, Earley CJ. RLS and blood donation. *Sleep Med*. 2009;10(8):844-849.

32. Winkelman JW, Chertow GM, Lazarus JM. Restless legs syndrome in end-stage renal disease. *Am J Kidney Dis*. 1996;28:372-378.

33. Kavanagh D, Siddiqui S, Geddes CC. Restless legs syndrome in patients on dialysis. *Am J Kidney Dis*. 2004;43:763-771.

34. Hui DS, Wong TY, Li TS, et al. Prevalence of sleep disturbances in Chinese patients with end stage renal failure on maintenance hemodialysis. *Med Sci Monit*. 2002;8:CR331-CR336.

35. Manconi M, Govoni V, De Vito A, et al. Restless legs syndrome and pregnancy. *Neurology*. 2004;63:1065-1069.

36. Tunc T, Karadag YS, Dogulu F, Inan LE. Predisposing factors of restless legs syndrome in pregnancy. *Mov Disord*. 2007; 22:627-631.

37. Salih AM, Gray RE, Mills KR, Webley M. A clinical, serological and neurophysiological study of restless legs syndrome in rheumatoid arthritis. *Br J Rheumatol*. 1994;33:60-63.

38. Prado GF, Allen RP, Trevisani VM, Toscano VG, Earley CJ. Sleep disruption in systemic sclerosis (scleroderma) patients: clinical and polysomnographic findings. *Sleep Med*. 2002;3:341-345.

39. Gudbjornsson B, Broman JE, Hetta J, Hallgren R. Sleep disturbances in patients with primary Sjogren's syndrome. *Br J Rheumatol*. 1993;32:1072-1076.

40. Yunus MB, Aldag JC. Restless legs syndrome and leg cramps in fibromyalgia syndrome: a controlled study. *BMJ*. 1996;312:1339.

41. Rutkove SB, Matheson JK, Logigian EL. Restless legs syndrome in patients with polyneuropathy. *Muscle Nerve*. 1996;19:670-672.

42. Gemignani F, Brindani F, Negrotti A, Vitetta F, Alfieri S, Marbini A. Restless legs syndrome and polyneuropathy. *Mov Disord*. 2006;21:1254-1257.

43. Gemignani F, Brindani F, Vitetta F, Marbini A, Calzetti S. Restless legs syndrome in diabetic neuropathy: a frequent manifestation of small fiber neuropathy. *J Peripher Nerv Syst*. 2007;12:50-53.

44. Lopes LA, Lins Cde M, Adeodato VG, et al. Restless legs syndrome and quality of sleep in type 2 diabetes. *Diabetes Care*. 2005;28:2633-2636.

45. Merlino G, Fratticci L, Valente M, et al. Association of restless legs syndrome in type 2 diabetes: a case-control study. *Sleep*. 2007;30(7):866-871.

46. Ondo WG, Vuong KD, Jankovic J. Exploring the relationship between Parkinson disease and restless legs syndrome. *Arch Neurol*. 2002;59:421-424.

47. Walters AS, Hickey K, Maltzman J, et al. A questionnaire study of 138 patients with restless legs syndrome: the 'Night-Walkers' survey. *Neurology*. 1996;46:92-95.

48. Ondo W, Jankovic J. Restless legs syndrome: clinicoetiologic correlates. *Neurology*. 1996;47:1435-1441.

49. Montplaisir J, Boucher S, Poirier G, Lavigne G, Lapierre O, Lesperance P. Clinical, polysomnographic, and genetic characteristics of restless legs syndrome: a study of 133 patients diagnosed with new standard criteria. *Mov Disord*. 1997;12:61-65.

50. Winkelmann J, Wetter TC, Collado-Seidel V, et al. Clinical characteristics and frequency of the hereditary restless legs syndrome in a population of 300 patients. *Sleep*. 2000;23:597-602.

51. Allen RP, La Buda MC, Becker P, Earley CJ. Family history study of the restless legs syndrome. *Sleep Med*. 2002; 3(suppl):S3-S7.

52. Winkelmann J, Muller-Myhsok B, Wittchen HU, et al. Complex segregation analysis of restless legs syndrome provides evidence for an autosomal dominant mode of inheritance in early age at onset families. *Ann Neurol*. 2002;52:297-302.

53. Mathias RA, Hening W, Washburn M, et al. Segregation analysis of restless legs syndrome: possible evidence for a major gene in a family study using blinded diagnoses. *Hum Hered*. 2006;62:157-164.

54. Winkelmann J, Lichtner P, Schormair B, et al. Variants in the neuronal nitric oxide synthase (nNOS, NOS1) gene are associated with restless legs syndrome. *Mov Disord*. 2008;23:350-358.

55. Winkelmann J, Schormair B, Lichtner P, et al. Genome-wide association study in restless legs syndrome identifies common variants in three genomic regions. *Nature Genet*. 2007;39(8):1000-1006.

56. Stefansson H, Rye DB, Hicks A, et al. A genetic risk factor for periodic limb movements in sleep. *N Engl J Med*. 2007; 357(7):639-647.

57. Schormair B, Kemlink D, Roeske D. et al. PTPRD9protein tyrosine phosphatase receptor type delta) is associated with restless legs syndrome. *Nat Genet*. 2008;40:946-948.

58. Kemlink D, Polo O, Frauscher B, et al. Replication of restless legs syndrome loci in three European populations. *J Med Genet*. 2009;46:315-318.

59. Hening W, Walters AS, Allen RP, Montplaisir J, Myers A, Ferini-Strambi L. Impact, diagnosis and treatment of restless legs syndrome (RLS) in a primary care population: the REST (RLS epidemiology, symptoms, and treatment) primary care study. *Sleep Med*. 2004;5:237-246.

60. Happe S, Vennemann M, Evers S, Berger K. Treatment wish of individuals with known and unknown restless legs syndrome in the community. *J Neurol*. 2008;255:1365-1371.

61. Allen RP, Earley CJ. Validation of the Johns Hopkins restless legs severity scale. *Sleep Med*. 2001;2:239-242.

62. Vahedi H, Kuchle M, Trenkwalder C, Krenz CJ. Peridural morphine administration in restless legs status. *Anasthesiol Intensivmed Notfallmed Schmerzther*. 1994;29:368-370.

63. Allen RP, Earley CJ. Defining the phenotype of the restless legs syndrome (RLS) using age-of-symptom-onset. *Sleep Med*. 2000;1:11-19.

64. Picchietti DL, England SJ, Walters AS, Willis K, Verrico T. Periodic limb movement disorder and restless legs syndrome in children with attention-deficit hyperactivity disorder. *J Child Neurol*. 1998;13(12):588-594.

65. Allen RP, Picchietti D, Hening WA, Trenkwalder C, Walters AS, Montplaisi J; Restless Legs Syndrome Diagnosis and Epidemiology workshop at the National Institutes of Health; International Restless Legs Syndrome Study Group. Restless legs syndrome: diagnostic criteria, special considerations, and epidemiology. A report from the restless legs syndrome diagnosis and epidemiology workshop at the National Institutes of Health. *Sleep Med*. 2003;4(2):101-119.

66. Walters AS, Picchietti DL, Ehrenberg BL, Wagner ML. Restless legs syndrome in childhood and adolescence. *Pediatr Neurol*. 1994;11(3):241-245.

67. Cortese S, Konofal E, Lecendreux M, et al. Restless legs syndrome and attention-deficit/hyperactivity disorder: a review of the literature. *Sleep*. 2005;28(8):1007-1013.

68. Walters AS. Is there a subpopulation of children with growing pains who really have Restless Legs Syndrome? A review of the literature. *Sleep Med*. 2002;3(2):93-98.

69. Rajaram SS, Walters AS, England SJ, Mehta D, Nizam F. Some children with growing pains may actually have restless legs syndrome. *Sleep*. 2004;27(4):767-773.

4 Pathophysiology

Nervous System Dysfunction

RLS is generally considered a neurologic disorder arising from the central nervous system (CNS). There has not been any evidence of specific lesion, neurodegeneration, or cell loss associated with RLS. Also, unlike other structurally based CNS conditions, RLS has not been associated with any other CNS-mediated functions other than disturbance in mood and, to a lesser degree, in cognition (eg, executive function). Therefore, it is likely that the etiology of RLS is due to CNS dysfunction at a cellular and functional level rather than due to structural CNS lesions. Nevertheless, it remains unclear where the RLS-related CNS alterations can be localized along the neuraxis, from spinal cord to cortex. In fact, there is even a suggestion that, at least in some patients, abnormalities of peripheral nerves may contribute to development of RLS (**Table 4.1**).

■ Electrophysiologic Studies

While not all studies are positive, several studies have suggested that there might be enhanced reflex activity in RLS, especially increases in late components of reflexes. This has been found for spinal flexion reflexes in both primary[1] and secondary RLS[2] and for startle reflexes (mediated by the reticulospinal tract).[3,4] Transcranial magnetic stimulation studies have found intact motor pathways, but evidence exists for decreased intracortical and subcortical inhibition, suggesting hyperexcitation due to diminished inhibition.[5-8] The reversal of these alterations with dopaminergic therapy has been demonstrated.[9,10]

TABLE 4.1 — Evidence for Involvement of Different Regions of the Nervous System in RLS

Peripheral Nerves
- Increased evidence of neuropathy in RLS patients[1,2]

Spinal Cord
- Presence of PLM in cord transected patients[3]
- Abnormal spinal reflexes in RLS[4]

Brain Stem
- Abnormal reticular formation and red nucleus activation during symptoms[5,6]

Cerebellum
- Abnormal cerebellar activation during symptoms[5]
- RLS in spinocerebellar ataxia[7]

Thalamus
- Increased pulvinar gray matter density[8]
- Striatal dopamine D_2-receptor involvement in RLS[9]

Basal Ganglia
- Autopsy studies show iron deficiency and protein abnormalities in substantia nigra[10,11]
- MRI and echo show reduced brain stem iron in RLS[12-15]

Cortex
- Imaging evidence of abnormal status of cortical pain areas[6,16]
- Magnetic stimulation demonstrates decreased intracortical inhibition[17,18]

1 Hattan E, et al. *Neurology*. 2009;72:955-960.
2 Polydefkis M, et al. *Neurology*. 2000;55:1115-1121.
3 Bara-Jimenez W, et al. *Neurology*. 2000;54:1609-1616.
4 Clemens S, et al. *Neurology*. 2006;67:125-130.
5 Bucher SF, et al. *Ann Neurol*. 1997;41:639-645
6 von Spiczak S, et al. *Brain*. 2005;128:906-917.
7 Schols L, et al. *Neurology*. 1998;51:1603-1607.
8 Etgen T, et al. *Neuroimage*. 2005;24:1242-1247.
9 Cervenka S, et al. *Brain*. 2006;129:2017-2028.
10 Wang X, et al. *J Neurol Sci*. 2004;220:59-66.
11 Connor JR, et al. *Neurology*. 2003;61:304-309.
12 Allen RP, et al. *Neurology*. 2001;56:263-265.
13 Earley CJ, et al. *Sleep Med*. 2006;7:458-461.
14 Schmidauer C, et al. *Ann Neurol*. 2005;58:630-634.
15 Godau J, et al. *Mov Disord*. 2007;22:187-192.
16 San Pedro EC, et al. *J Rheumatol*. 1998;25:2270-2275.
17 Tergau FS, et al. *Neurology*. 1999;53:861-864.
18 Scalise A, et al. *Sleep*. 2006;29:770-775.

■ Imaging Studies

General studies of brain structure[11] and resting metabolism[12] have found no abnormalities in RLS. One functional magnetic resonance imaging (fMRI) study found abnormal bilateral cerebellar and thalamic activation during sensory symptoms, with additional red nucleus and reticular formation activity during periodic limb movements in wake (PLMW).[11] A single-photon emission computed tomography (SPECT) study of an affected parent/child pair showed changes consistent with pain (decreased caudate and increase anterior cingulate blood flow).[13] A positron emission tomography (PET) study using an opioid ligand found that there was altered activity in brain regions associated with the medial pain system (especially orbitofrontal cortex and anterior cingulate).[14] One MRI study found bilateral increases in gray matter in the pulvinar nucleus of the thalamus,[15] but this was not confirmed in drug-naïve subjects.[16] In fact, more recent studies could not replicate the previous findings of structural brain changes in RLS.[17,18] Dopamine-related PET neuroimaging studies are discussed in a later section.

■ Circadian Rhythms

The overall circadian rhythm is regulated by the suprachiasmatic nucleus of the hypothalamus, keeping many body functions cycling within a period of around 24 hours.[19,20] It has been established that all RLS symptoms also have a circadian rhythm with peak activity between the late evening and early morning (approximately 21:00 to 4:00 hours).[21-23] This period largely coincides with the daily rise in melatonin secretion, a key biologic marker of the intrinsic circadian clock.[24] The link between melatonin and RLS is not clear but may represent merely multiple effects of a general circadian process or might indicate some specific influence of melatonin on RLS. In fact, a recent study that administered exogenous melatonin to RLS patients found exacerbation of RLS symptoms reflected by increased suggested immobilization test (SIT) index.[25]

In summary, a variety of studies have suggested that while no discrete CNS lesion has been found in RLS, there may be altered function at various levels of the CNS.[26] The peripheral nervous system may also influence the development or expression of symptoms. However, these studies have not yet revealed what is the key locus or loci in causing RLS. There may be more clues from examining altered neurotransmitter and metabolic systems in RLS.

Neurotransmitter Systems

■ Dopamine and CNS Iron

The connection of RLS to the dopamine system has been established by the response of RLS to dopaminergic treatments in almost all studies performed to date. After the publication of initial studies that reported the invariably positive response of RLS to dopamine agonist,[27-29] RLS, like PD, was hypothesized to be a disorder due to decreased brain dopamine storage and possible neurodegeneration. Some imaging studies supported the dopamine depletion hypothesis by reporting a decrease in dopamine markers,[30] but conflicting findings exist.[31] One imaging study reported that D_2 receptors were increased both within and without the striatum.[32] Overall, previous studies based on PET and SPECT studies of dopamine-2/3 receptor (D2R) binding potential (BP) have shown inconsistent results.[33] A recent PET-based studies on dopamine transporter in RLS subjects found significant decreased in DAT binding potentials and suggested that membrane-bound striatal DAT, but not total cellular DAT, may be decreased in RLS.[34]

Another possible abnormality concerning dopamine could be an altered amplitude of its circadian rhythm.[35-37] Cerebrospinal fluid (CSF) studies have found that dopamine metabolites show greater circadian variation in RLS patients than in controls.[38] RLS patients may have as much dopamine as others—perhaps even more at certain phases of the daily cycle—

but the variation may induce symptoms selectively at certain times of day. This effect may explain one endocrine study that found that administered levodopa selectively produced enhanced endocrine responses when administered to patients in the evening.[39]

One hypothesis that may provide a mechanism for such dopamine abnormalities is the idea that in many cases, RLS is induced by inadequate levels of CNS iron.[40-43] Several lines of evidence for this concept are listed in **Table 4.2**. The basic hypothesis (**Figure 4.1**) is that either through altered cellular mechanisms or depressed body stores, the iron levels in dopaminergic neurons drop (**Figure 4.2**). As a consequence, neuronal function changes and the result may be disruption of synaptic function[44] or accentuation of the circadian rhythm of dopamine.[45] Under this concept, those with familial, genetically based RLS is hypothesized to have a tendency toward depressed uptake and retention of brain iron, while those with secondary RLS would have conditions in which body iron stores are depleted, thereby drawing out iron from the brain. While this CNS iron model of RLS is promising, several key details of this model remain elusive and the model needs to be tested further to explain the etiopathogenesis of RLS.

So far studies of brain iron deficiencies in humans with RLS have focused on the substantia nigra, the key nucleus for parkinsonian pathology. However, voluntary motor function is normal in most RLS patients.[46] Animal-model studies have generally concentrated on the A11 dopamine system, a diffuse and hard-to-study cell grouping that sends dopaminergic axons down to the spinal cord.[47] To date, it has not been conclusively shown that disrupting the A11 system produces a suitable model for RLS, and studies on the human A11 system have not been done. We are therefore still unsure which dopaminergic system is most responsible for RLS.

TABLE 4.2 — Evidence for the Iron-Dopamine Hypothesis for Causation of RLS

Iron Deficiency Is Associated With RLS

Prominent Secondary RLS Conditions Are Associated With Iron Deficiency
- Pregnancy
- Anemia
- Uremia
- Rheumatoid arthritis

CSF Findings
- RLS patients show decreased CSF levels of iron storage marker (ferritin) and increased transferrin
- RLS patients show strong circadian rhythm of dopamine metabolites and related compounds[1]

Brain Iron Levels
- In vivo studies show low brain stem iron
- Autopsy studies show low levels of iron in substantia nigra neurons with decreased ferritin and increased transferrin[2]
- Autopsy studies show abnormalities of iron regulating proteins consistent with decreased transferrin receptor in the face of low iron[3]
- Autopsy studies show that there are alterations in the brain iron management protein profile in RLS compared with controls at the site of blood-brain interface[4]

Altered Dopamine-System Autopsy Findings in Iron Deficient RLS Patients
- Decreased thy-1 synaptic adhesion protein
- Increased tyrosine hydroxylase, dopamine, and dopamine metabolites

Animal Models
- A11 spinal dopamine tract lesion creates rodents with behavioral similarities to RLS[5,6]
- Feeding iron-deficient diet enhances RLS-like behaviors[7]

[1] Earley CJ, et al. *Sleep Med*. 2006;7:263-268.
[2] Connor JR, et al. *Neurology*. 2003;61:304-309.
[3] Connor JR, et al. *Neurology*. 2004;62:1563-1567.
[4] Connor JR, et al. *Brain*. 2011;134:959-968.
[5] Clemens S, et al. *Neurology*. 2006;67:125-130.
[6] Lopes C, et al. *Mov Disord*. 2012;27:413-420.
[7] Ondo WG, et al. *Sleep Med*. 2007;8:344-348.

FIGURE 4.1 — Overall Model of Iron and Dopamine Causing RLS

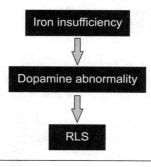

The model stresses that the primary deficit is in reduced iron levels that then cause abnormalities in dopamine-system functioning. A major support for the hypothesis is the therapeutic benefit obtained regularly with dopamine and sometimes with iron supplementation.

Other Systems

The endogenous opiate system has been implicated in RLS by the favorable response of patients to a wide variety of opioid medications.[48-51] Imaging studies have also suggested that RLS symptoms are correlated with activity or binding changes in pain-relevant CNS structures.[13,14] One early case study provided some evidence that RLS might act through the dopamine system,[52] but strong opioids have been found to be effective even when dopamine agents have failed or have caused iatrogenic exacerbation of RLS (augmentation).[51] Reversal of therapeutic effect by opioid blockers (naloxone) does indicate that the effect is specific to the endogenous opiate system.[53] The exact role of opioids and the relation between the opiate and dopamine systems remain areas for further exploration.

FIGURE 4.2 — Midbrain Stained for Iron in RLS Patient and Control

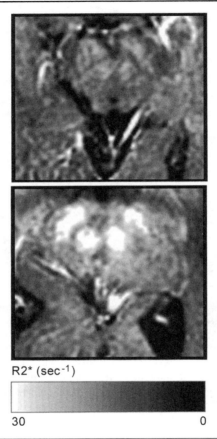

R2* (sec⁻¹)

30   0

R2* magnetic resonance images in a 70-year-old, RLS patient *(top)* and a 71-year-old, control subject *(bottom)*. Much lower R2* relaxation rates are apparent in the RLS case in both red nucleus and substantia nigra, indicating lower iron content.

Allen RP, et al. *Neurology*. 2001;56:263-265.

Other neuronal systems—the adrenergic, serotoninergic, glutaminergic, gabaergic, orexinergic, histaminergic, and adenosinergic—have been implicated by some therapeutic or other studies in RLS, but evidence for and understanding of their potential roles is only at an early stage. Given the complex interrelationships of neural systems in the brain, it is likely that many systems may play some role in modulating the development, expression, and perception of RLS symptoms.

4

REFERENCES

1. Bara-Jimenez W, Hallett M. Increased spinal cord excitability in patients with restless legs syndrome. *Mov Disord*. 1998; 13(suppl 2):294.

2. Aksu M, Bara-Jimenez W. State dependent excitability changes of spinal flexor reflex in patients with restless legs syndrome secondary to chronic renal failure. *Sleep Med*. 2002;3:427-430.

3. Frauscher B, Loscher WN, Hogl B, Poewe W, Kofler M. Auditory startle reaction is disinhibited in idiopathic restless legs syndrome. *Sleep*. 2007;30:489-493.

4. Rijsman RM, Stam CJ, de Weerd AW. Abnormal H-reflexes in periodic limbmovment disorder: impact on understanding the pathophysiology of the disorder. *Clin Neurophysiol*. 2005;116:204-210.

5. Tergau F, Wischer S, Paulus W. Motor system excitability in patients with restless legs syndrome. *Neurology*. 1999;52:1060-1063.

6. Stiasny-Kolster K, Haeske H, Tergau F, Muller HH, Braune HJ, Oertel WH. Cortical silent period is shortened in restless legs syndrome independently from circadian rhythm. *Suppl Clin Neurophysiol*. 2003;56:381-389.

7. Scalise A, Cadore IP, Gigli GL. Motor cortex excitability in restless legs syndrome. *Sleep Med*. 2004;5:393-396.

8. Scalise A, Pittaro-Cadore I, Golob EJ, Gigli GL. Absence of postexercise and delayed facilitation of motor cortex excitability in restless legs syndrome: evidence of altered cortical plasticity? *Sleep*. 2006;29:770-775.

9. Nardone R, Ausserer H, Bratti A, et al. Cabergoline reverses cortical hyperexcitability in patients with restless legs syndrome. *Acta Neurol Scand*. 2006;114:244-249.

10. Scalise A, Pittaro-Cadore I, Janes F, Marinig R, Gigli GL. Changes of cortical excitability after dopaminergic treatment in restless legs syndrome. *Sleep Med*. 2010;11:75-81.

11. Bucher SF, Seelos KC, Oertel WH, Reiser M, Trenkwalder C. Cerebral generators involved in the pathogenesis of the restless legs syndrome. *Ann Neurol*. 1997;41:639-645.

12. Trenkwalder C, Walters AS, Hening WA, et al. Positron emission tomographic studies in restless legs syndrome. *Mov Disord*. 1999;14:141-145.

13. San Pedro EC, Mountz JM, Mountz JD, Liu HG, Katholi CR, Deutsch G. Familial painful restless legs syndrome correlates with pain dependent variation of blood flow to the caudate, thalamus, and anterior cingulate gyrus. *J Rheumatol.* 1998;25:2270-2275.

14. von Spiczak S, Whone AL, Hammers A, et al. The role of opioids in restless legs syndrome: an [11C]diprenorphine PET study. *Brain.* 2005;128:906-917.

15. Etgen T, Draganski B, Ilg C, et al. Bilateral thalamic gray matter changes in patients with restless legs syndrome. *Neuroimage.* 2005;24:1242-1247.

16. Hornyak M, Ahrendts JC, Spiegelhalder K, et al. Voxel-based morphometry in unmedicated patients with restless legs syndrome. *Sleep Med.* 2007;9:22-26.

17. Comley RA, Cervenka S, Palhagen SE, et al. A comparison of gray mater density in restless legs syndrome patients and matched controls using voxel-based morphometry. *J Neuroimaging.* 2012;1:28-32.

18. Celle S, Roche F, Peyron R, et al. Lack of specific gray matter alterations in restless legs syndrome in elderly subjects. *J Neurol.* 2010;257:344-348.

19. Saper CB, Lu J, Chou TC, Gooley J. The hypothalamic integrator for circadian rhythms. *Trends Neurosci.* 2005;28:152-157.

20. Schibler U. Circadian time keeping: the daily ups and downs of genes, cells, and organisms. *Prog Brain Res.* 2006;153:271-282.

21. Hening WA, Walters AS, Wagner M, et al. Circadian rhythm of motor restlessness and sensory symptoms in the idiopathic restless legs syndrome. *Sleep.* 1999;22:901-912.

22. Trenkwalder C, Hening WA, Walters AS, Campbell SS, Rahman K, Chokroverty S. Circadian rhythm of periodic limb movements and sensory symptoms of restless legs syndrome. *Mov Disord.* 1999;14:102-110.

23. Michaud M, Dumont M, Paquet J, Desautels A, Fantini ML, Montplaisir J. Circadian variation of the effects of immobility on symptoms of restless legs syndrome. *Sleep.* 2005;28:843-846.

24. Michaud M, Dumont M, Selmaoui B, Paquet J, Fantini ML, Montplaisir J. Circadian rhythm of restless legs syndrome: relationship with biological markers. *Ann Neurol.* 2004;55:372-380.

4

25. Whittom S, Dumont M, Petit D, et al. Effect of melatonin and bright light administration on motor and sensory symptoms of RLS. *Sleep Med.* 2010;11:351-355.

26. Trenkwalder C, Paulus W. Restless legs syndrome: pathophysiology, clinical presentation and management. *Nat Rev Neurol.* 2010;6:337-346.

27. Akpinar S. Treatment of restless legs syndrome with levodopa plus benserazide. *Arch Neurol.* 1982;39:739.

28. Montplaisir J, Godbout R, Poirier G, Bedard MA. Restless legs syndrome and periodic movements in sleep: physiopathology and treatment with L-dopa. *Clin Neuropharmacol.* 1986;9:456-463.

29. Walters AS, Hening WA, Kavey N, Chokroverty S, Gidro-Frank S. A double-blind randomized crossover trial of bromocriptine and placebo in restless legs syndrome. *Ann Neurol.* 1988;24:455-458.

30. Turjanski N, Lees AJ, Brooks DJ. Striatal dopaminergic function in restless legs syndrome: 18F-dopa and 11C-raclopride PET studies. *Neurology.* 1999;52:932-937.

31. Eisensehr I, Wetter TC, Linke R, et al. Normal IPT and IBZM SPECT in drug-naive and levodopa-treated idiopathic restless legs syndrome. *Neurology.* 2001;57:1307-1309.

32. Cervenka S, Palhagen SE, Comley RA, et al. Support for dopaminergic hypoactivity in restless legs syndrome: a PET study on D2-receptor binding. *Brain.* 2006;129:2017-2028.

33. Trenkwalder C, Earley CJ. Neuroimaging in restless legs syndrome. In: Hening WA, Allen RP, Chokroverty S, Earley CJ, eds. *Restless Legs Syndrome.* Philadelphia, PA: Saunders Elsevier; 2009:78-82.

34. Earley CJ, Kuwabara H, Wong DF, et al. The dopamine transporter is decreased in the striatum of subjects with resistless legs syndrome. *Sleep.* 2011;34:341-347.

35. Davila R, Zumarraga M, Andia I, Friedhoff AJ. Persistence of cyclicity of the plasma dopamine metabolite, homovanillic acid, in neuroleptic treated schizophrenic patients. *Life Sci.* 1989;44:1117-1121.

36. Doran AR, Pickar D, Labarca R, et al. Evidence for a daily rhythm of plasma HVA in normal controls but not in schizophrenic patients. *Psychopharmacol Bull.* 1985;21:694-697.

37. Kawano Y, Kawasaki T, Kawazoe N, et al. Circadian variations of urinary dopamine, norepinephrine, epinephrine and sodium in normotensive and hypertensive subjects. *Nephron.* 1990;55:277-282.

38. Earley CJ, Hyland K, Allen RP. Circadian changes in CSF dopaminergic measures in restless legs syndrome. *Sleep Med.* 2006;7:263-268.

39. Garcia-Borreguero D, Larrosa O, Granizo JJ, de la Llave Y, Hening WA. Circadian variation in neuroendocrine response to L-dopa in patients with restless legs syndrome. *Sleep.* 2004; 27:669-673.

40. Earley CJ, Hyland K, Allen RP. Circadian changes in CSF dopaminergic measures in restless legs syndrome. *Sleep Med.* 2006;7:263-268.

41. Allen RP, Earley CJ. The role of iron in restless legs syndrome. *Mov Disord.* 2007;22(suppl 18):S440-S448.

42. Allen R. Dopamine and iron in the pathophysiology of restless legs syndrome (RLS). *Sleep Med.* 2004;5:385-391.

43. Astrakas LG, Konitsiotis S, Marganti P, Tsouli S, Tzarouhi L, Argyropoulou MI. T2 relaxometry and fMRI of the brain in late-onset restless legs syndrome. *Neurology.* 2008;16:911-916.

44. Wang X, Wiesinger J, Beard J, et al. Thy1 expression in the brain is affected by iron and is decreased in Restless Legs Syndrome. *J Neurol Sci.* 2004;220:59-66.

45. Dean T Jr, Allen RP, O'Donnell CP, Earley CJ. The effects of dietary iron deprivation on murine circadian sleep architecture. *Sleep Med.* 2006;7:634-640.

46. Alberts JL, Adler CH, Saling M, Stelmach GE. Prehension patterns in restless legs syndrome patients. *Parkinsonism Relat Disord.* 2001;7:143-148.

47. Clemens S, Rye D, Hochman S. Restless legs syndrome: revisiting the dopamine hypothesis from the spinal cord perspective. *Neurology.* 2006;67:125-130.

48. Walters AS, Wagner ML, Hening WA, et al. Successful treatment of the idiopathic restless legs syndrome in a randomized double-blind trial of oxycodone versus placebo. *Sleep.* 1993;16:327-332.

49. Walters AS, Winkelmann J, Trenkwalder C, et al. Long-term follow-up on restless legs syndrome patients treated with opioids. *Mov Disord.* 2001;16:1105-1109.

50. Vignatelli L, Billiard M, Clarenbach P, et al. EFNS guidelines on management of restless legs syndrome and periodic limb movement disorder in sleep. *Eur J Neurol.* 2006;13:1049-1065.

51. Ondo WG. Methadone for refractory restless legs syndrome. *Mov Disord.* 2005;20:345-348.

4

52. Montplaisir J, Lorrain D, Godbout R. Restless legs syndrome and periodic leg movements in sleep: the primary role of dopaminergic mechanism. *Eur Neurol*. 1991;31:41-43.

53. Walters A, Hening W, Cote L, Fahn S. Dominantly inherited restless legs with myoclonus and periodic movements of sleep: a syndrome related to the endogenous opiates? *Adv Neurol*. 1986;43:309-319.

5 Consequences

RLS has a myriad of consequences, especially for patients with moderate to severe symptoms. It has significant effects on sleep, energy/vitality, daily activities, behavior, cognition, and mood and subsequently causes social, occupation, educational and other important areas of functioning, and reduces quality of life. The most significant and noticeable consequence is its impact on sleep. In addition, several other unique aspects of RLS create havoc in the life of RLS sufferers.

Impact on Sleep

■ Difficulty Getting to Sleep

Bedtime tends to be the most difficult time for patients with moderate to severe RLS. The bothersome RLS symptoms typically peak at bedtime and often prevent RLS suffers from falling asleep. Once lying in bed, RLS symptoms tend to exacerbate dramatically and force sufferers to move their affected limbs or get out of bed and walk to relieve their uncomfortable urge to move. Patients with RLS often refer to themselves as "night walkers," which also is the name of the quarterly newsletter published by the RLS Foundation.[1]

The REST General Population Study[1] (which interviewed >16,000 adults in the United States, France, Germany, Italy, Spain, and the UK) found that 75.5% of the RLS sufferers (people reporting moderately to severely distressing RLS symptoms at least twice weekly) reported at least one sleep-related symptom. About 48% of these RLS sufferers reported an inability to fall asleep. Similarly, the REST Primary Care Study[2] (which investigated >23,000 patients from the practices of 182 primary care physicians in the United States, France, Germany, Spain, and the UK) found that 68.6% of RLS sufferers took 30 minutes or longer than the RLS-free participants to fall asleep (**Figure 5.1**).

Unlike people with other medical problems who cannot fall asleep, those with RLS often cannot simply go to another bed or a comfortable place to try to fall asleep or even rest. People with milder and intermittent forms of RLS may not have significant problems falling asleep. They may report occasional difficulty falling asleep but, in general, sleep is not a major complaint in this group. In contrast, for those with severe RLS, their irresistible, uncomfortable urge to move their legs (and other affected body parts) force them to become "night walkers." This nightly torment that sometimes lasts for hours or even all night has been aptly described as torture.

Many RLS patients whose symptoms are relieved by treatment may continue to have problems falling asleep. After years of disrupted sleeping patterns due to RLS symptoms, RLS sufferers often develop abnormal sleeping patterns, such as being conditioned to delay falling asleep until early morning. Therefore, clinicians may have to treat them for persistent insomnia even after the RLS symptoms have been completely resolved.

■ Difficulty in Maintaining Sleep

The REST primary care study[2] also showed that RLS sufferers have difficulty maintaining sleep. They found that 60.1% of this group woke up three or more times per night (**Figure 5.2**). The RLS sufferers often have a hard time falling asleep after these intermittent awakenings due to their recurring RLS symptoms. Sleep deprivation from their inability to fall asleep and maintain proper sleep can take a toll on quality of life and often results in further daytime RLS-related consequences as discussed below.

FIGURE 5.1 — Time to Fall Asleep for RLS Sufferers: REST Study

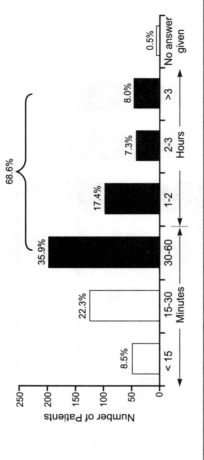

Hening WA, et al. *Sleep Med.* 2004;5:237-246.

FIGURE 5.2 — The Impact of RLS on Awakenings at Night: REST Study

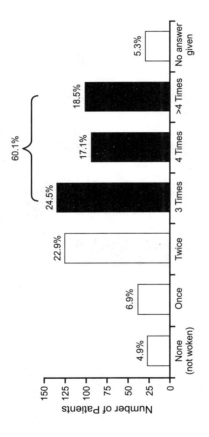

Hening WA, et al. *Sleep Med.* 2004;5:237-246.

The effect of sleep deprivation from both sleep-onset and sleep-maintenance insomnia described above can be substantial. When combined with the inability to rest during the daytime (for those with more severe RLS), the RLS sufferers can have significant disruptions in their lifestyle and daily activities.

■ **Fatigue and Daytime Sleepiness**

The REST primary care study[2] found that 60.1% of RLS sufferers reported that they lacked energy when experiencing RLS symptoms and 57.2% of this group stated that their daily activities were disturbed. Another study[3] found that 61% of RLS patients studied had increased sleepiness assessed by the Epworth Sleepiness Scale and increased fatigue assessed by Fatigue Severity Scale. Furthermore, the above studies and an additional one in 2004[4] found RLS sufferers to have a decrease in their energy/vitality scores on the Short Form 36 Health Survey (SF-36). One recent study even demonstrated that increased daytime sleepiness was directly associated to more frequent RLS symptoms.[5] On occasion, the inability to sleep at nighttime may be so severe that the patient may walk most of the night or fall asleep only while standing. This somnambulant behavior presents health and safety risks exemplified by one case report about a patient whose RLS symptoms resulted in repeated falls causing multiple skeletal fractures.[6]

Complaints of daytime fatigue are very common in RLS sufferers. Despite battling these symptoms, many do try to lead full, normal lives. Interestingly, despite daytime fatigue and sleepiness, there has been no report of association between RLS and increased risk for motor vehicle accidents as might be expected. It might be that bothersome RLS symptoms, which tend to increase while driving, prevent the onset of sleep. For the same reason, it is often difficult for people with RLS to nap during the daytime despite their sleep deprivation.

■ **Concentration and Cognition**

The sleep deprivation described can account for significant problems with concentration and in cognition. The resulting fatigue, coupled with the intrusion of bothersome RLS symptoms, provides understanding of the mental fogginess experienced by RLS patients. Not many studies have yet examined this issue, but the REST general population study found that 19.2% of RLS sufferers reported difficulty concentrating in the afternoon, and 17.5%, the next evening after not sleeping well.

A recent study[7] that specifically examined cognitive deficits associated with moderate to severe RLS found similar sizeable deficits, especially with verbal fluency, to those reported losing a full night of sleep. Ironically, the same research group found that RLS sufferers actually performed better than the sleep-restricted controls on pre-frontal lobe specific cognitive test.[8] More detailed discussion on the impact of RLS on cognition is on *Chapter 12*.

Impact on Mood

Many studies have found high prevalence of depression and anxiety symptoms in RLS patients.[1-5,9-10] It is thought that the chronic discomfort of RLS symptoms (similar to that of any other chronic pain disorder) and chronic insomnia lead to depression.[11] A recent study demonstrated a dose-dependent relationship between RLS symptom frequency and self-reported depression and anxiety outcomes.[5] Another study[10] reported that most patients developed their anxiety or depression after the onset of RLS symptoms, suggesting that depression may occur because of the RLS symptoms. However, it is not yet completely clear whether the association between RLS and mood disorders are due to a symptomatic epiphenomenon or shared pathophysiologic mechanism between RLS and mood disorder.

Nevertheless, there is little doubt that depression and anxiety are strongly associated with RLS and frequent complaints among RLS patients as the association of depression and RLS has been made repeatedly in the medical literature.[9] Similarly, depression and anxiety disorder patients also frequently complain about RLS-like symptoms. Adding complexity to the elucidation of this relationship is the fact that many CNS-acting medications prescribed to treat depression and anxiety are likely to worsen RLS symptoms. In 2013, RLS is scheduled to be elevated to its own diagnostic category in the DSM-5. The psychiatric aspect of RLS is explored in greater detail in *Chapter 12*.

Impact on Cardiovascular Health

Several recent studies have demonstrated a marked decrease in general health in people with RLS.[1-4,9] The SF-36 scores in these studies reveal significantly decreased quality of life very similar to that of other chronic disorders (such as depression, chronic obstructive pulmonary disease, osteoarthritis, diabetes, congestive heart failure, etc). In addition, the general health, bodily pain, and physical functioning role parameters are universally decreased. This disease has a marked impact on the life of RLS patients.

There is a growing body of evidence that suggests associations between RLS and various cardiovascular risk factors such as diabetes, hypertension, obesity, dyslipidemia, and others.[12] The Wisconsin Sleep Cohort study[5] found a cross-sectional association of RLS symptoms with cardiovascular disease similar to that in a previous study in Sweden.[13] More recently, the Sleep Heart Health Study reported that odds ratio for coronary heart disease was 2.05 (95% CI: 1.38 to 3.04) and cardiovascular disease was 2.07 (95% CI: 1.43 to 3.00).[14] These cross-sectional findings were subsequently followed by a longitudinal study that reported higher risk of developing nonfatal myocardial infarction (RR: 1.80; 95% CI: 1.07-3.01) for nonfatal myocardial infarction and fatal CHD (RR: 1.49; 95% CI: 0.55-4.04) among women with RLS for 3 years or longer, relative to women without RLS.[15] The cause of these associations remains speculative, but sympathetic overactivity associated with RLS/PLMS, as manifested by increased pulse rate and blood pressure coincident with PLMS, suggest a potential biologic mechanism underlying this relationship. A recent review by Walters and colleagues hypothesizes the three potential pathways: 1) the sympathetic hyperactivity associated with RLS/PLMS may lead to daytime hypertension and subsequent heart disease and stroke; 2) sympathetic hyperactivity associated with RLS/PLMS could lead to atherosclerotic plaque formation and rupture; and 3) comorbidities associated with RLS/PLMS, such as renal failure, diabetes, iron deficiency, and insomnia, could lead to heart disease and stroke.[16]

Avocational Impairment

RLS can prevent people from enjoying social activities in life. All sedentary situations, particularly during the evenings, could seem troublesome; therefore, activities that limit movements are often avoided.

■ Social Events

Religious services, social meetings (eg, theater, book clubs, lectures, etc), and evenings with friends or family are often on the list of things to be avoided. The more formal activities such attendance at church services are especially difficult as fidgety movement or walking during the service are socially inappropriate. However, even during more informal, evening get-together with friends or family, the urge to move and walk around while others are sitting quietly may seem embarrassing to the RLS sufferer.

In addition, the fatigue, sleepiness, and inability to concentrate are common experiences among RLS sufferers and prevent them from enjoying these social events. Therefore, many RLS sufferers shun them and make up excuses (usually not referring to their RLS since most people neither understand RLS nor empathize with RLS sufferers) to avoid them.

Theaters and movies might pose less of a threat to the RLS sufferers because the anonymity associated with these activities seems more protective to them than gathering among friends and family. However, the long duration of sedentary inactivity while watching plays or movies may be difficult to tolerate for RLS sufferers. For example, while at a late-evening opera, many who suffer the bedtime RLS symptoms will find their symptoms gradually escalate during the final act and eventually prevent them from hearing the closing arias.

Some coping mechanisms could enable those with RLS to go to the movies or theater. Sitting in an aisle seat or on the back row may facilitate movement or going for a quick walk to relieve symptoms. It may be possible to walk and view the performance from behind a glass at the back of the auditorium. However, many RLS patients feel that the effort and stigma of relieving their symptoms in public are just not worth it and tend to avoid these venues altogether.

Relationships With Friends and Family

Relationships tend to be a problem for those with significant RLS problems. The lifestyle restrictions due to RLS often prevent RLS sufferers from forming and maintaining close relationships.

■ Family and Friends

The relationships with family and friends are often sustained and cemented by sharing common activities, such as watching TV, taking trips, going to movies or attending church activities, sitting and talking while at meals, etc. For RLS sufferers, these sedentary activities are hard to cope with and often avoided. Also, fatigue and lack of energy due to sleepless nights also take away the energy for the RLS sufferers to participate in these activities.

Even when the RLS sufferers resolve to participate in such events through willpower, their family and friends might get tired of hearing the repeated excuses and might assume that the RLS sufferer is a loner who does not like to socialize. Many RLS sufferers feel socially isolated and feel ostracized by their friends and family. Anxiety and depression that are common among RLS sufferers could lead to further social withdrawal and limit their opportunities to bond with others even further.

People with RLS become frustrated with their friends and family as they hear over and over again, "But you don't look like you have a medical condition; you look well enough to go out with us tonight!" As the RLS symptoms do not have any serious-appearing external manifestations (except for the person walking, rubbing the affected area of leg, kicking), this disorder is usually not taken very seriously by friends and family. The excuse of RLS is often interpreted as just not wanting to be with or do things with the friends and family members.

■ Intimacy (Spousal/Bed Partner Issues)

Dating can be a problem for similar reasons that were previously described. However, becoming intimate and sharing a bed presents even more difficulties for RLS sufferers. Bedtime is when RLS symptoms tend to peak, thereby making it difficult to rest in bed. The spouse or bed partner of an RLS sufferer can easily get annoyed at the continued movements necessary to relieve RLS symptoms. Once asleep, PLM may disturb the bed partner or even cause them injury.

Not being able to sleep with the bed partner is often misperceived as not wanting to sleep with them and easily results in hurt feelings. There are many anecdotal reports of this misunderstanding leading to the breakup of couples or even marriages. The loss of the ability to share a bed with your partner is one of the major complaints of those afflicted with RLS. It is bad enough that they must endure the social isolation due to unintended problems in maintaining relationships with family and friends. Furthermore, they may lose the intimacy and support of their spouse or partner.

Occupational Consequences

Just as RLS impacts other facets of daily life, RLS often impacts work negatively. Any occupation that requires sedentary activities is prone to be problematic for RLS sufferers. Sometimes these RLS-related impediments to performing a job can be avoided. However, many types of employment are not as flexible and may thus not be suitable for those with RLS.

■ Impact on Job Performance and Selection

Any occupation that includes desk work, long meetings, driving long distances, or other sedentary tasks is stressful for most RLS patients. This limitation clearly eliminates a substantial proportion of appropriate workplaces for RLS sufferers and narrows the scope of work that is suitable for people with RLS in the already tight job market.

That does not mean that anyone with RLS should quit their job once they develop RLS while employed. There are often ways to work around the problem (discussed later) that may help the person sustain good job performance. Cooperation of fellow employees and management is usually helpful and often necessary. It is easy to imagine how a patient with moderate to severe RLS may not be able to sit long hours at a desk or sit with peers or clients during long meetings.

The choice of career may be important to people with RLS. If daytime RLS symptoms are interfering with performance despite treatment, a different type of job may be preferred. For example, a nurse or schoolteacher may do well despite RLS, as their work is conducive to walking whenever necessary and has only a small sedentary component in their daily duty. However, being promoted to administration with the associated desk work and meetings may be a career-ending promotion.

Shift work may also be problematic for some but may work for others. If the work is not sedentary, it may be appropriate, even for the peak RLS hours, as long as it allows for adequate sleep time at a later time. RLS patients who do not get enough sleep (which is common among shift workers) will develop more problems with their RLS symptoms. Shift work should be avoided unless it meets the requirements previously noted.

Some people with RLS prefer to be self-employed as they can choose their working hours, the amount of sedentary work, and even change their work environment to adjust to their unique RLS-related requirements.

Even with an RLS-friendly job, the performance of those with RLS may be poor. As noted, fatigue, daytime sleepiness, and problems with concentration and thinking may easily impair job performance. Problems with anxiety and depression may further impair the individual from functioning at work and interacting effectively with their coworkers. Inadequate treatment of RLS may easily result in poor job ratings, decreased income, and even loss of employment. Furthermore, some of the drugs used for RLS may cause daytime sleepiness and, despite helping RLS, may result in impairing work performance.

■ Disability

Those suffering from severe RLS may not be able to maintain their employment if their RLS symptoms deteriorate. For example, an RLS sufferer who cannot sit still to eat meals due to severe RLS symptoms might not be able to hold a sedentary desk job. Even for those who have occupations that do not require them to be sedentary, fatigue, daytime sleepiness, decreased concentration and mentation, anxiety, and depression associated with RLS might prevent them from performing their job duties adequately.

Thus it may be appropriate for some people with severe RLS to go on disability. Obtaining disability, however, even for those with more accepted and traditional illnesses, is often difficult. RLS presents additional hurdles as unrecognized medical condition by the Social Security Administration and related government agency. Also, the medical personnel who assess the level of disability for various medical conditions generally are not familiar with RLS. Therefore, the disability due to RLS is generally filed under the resultant medical consequence of RLS rather than the disorder itself.

If the RLS and PLM are causing excessive daytime sleepiness, objective measures, such as an overnight sleep study, multiple sleep latency test, or maintenance of wakefulness test, may provide objective evidence to document the degree of disability due to RLS. Physicians can be instrumental in assisting the RLS patient in obtaining approval for their disability. Proper documentation of the nature and extent of the disability can be critical in such cases. Although many people with disability eventually obtain approval, this process can take an inordinate amount of time. In general, RLS sufferers receive disability benefits only after careful documentation and advocacy by their health care providers.

Impact on Travel

In our modern, fast-paced world, those who do not suffer RLS tend to take travel for granted. Even people with more certain physical disabilities (eg, those who are wheelchair-bound) are accustomed to special accommodations that are legally required to ensure their safe traveling. The most difficult traveling situation for RLS sufferers is long airplane trips. Once the seatbelt sign illuminates (for take-off, turbulent weather, etc), they are simply trapped in their worst possible situation. There is simply no way to walk off the RLS symptoms, which rapidly escalate due to the compelled confinement and inactivity in the narrow airplane passenger seat. There are some methods of ameliorating this issue and they will be discussed in the chapters on treating RLS.

When possible, RLS sufferers generally prefer other modes of transportation than air travel. Trains are generally better tolerated as one can get up and walk whenever necessary. Buses, however, are more problematic for RLS sufferers as there is only a little aisle space in which to walk. Travel by sailing boat could be fine, but only if the size of the boat is large enough to allow enough movements for the passenger with RLS. Automobile trips are feasible as long as the RLS sufferer makes a frequent stops for walks. Longer trips can be harder or even impossible for those with more severe RLS.

REFERENCES

1. Allen RP, Walters AS, Montplaisir J, et al. Restless legs syndrome prevalence and impact: REST general population study. *Arch Intern Med.* 2005;165:1286-1292.

2. Hening W, Walters AS, Allen RP, Montplaisir J, Myers A, Ferini-Strambi L. Impact, diagnosis and treatment of restless legs syndrome (RLS) in a primary care population: the REST (RLS epidemiology, symptoms, and treatment) primary care study. *Sleep Med.* 2004;5:237-246.

3. Gerhard R, Bosse A, Uzun D, Orth M, Kotterba S. Quality of life in restless legs syndrome. Influence of daytime sleepiness and fatigue [in German]. *Med Klin (Munich).* 2005; 100(11):704-709.

4. Abetz L, Allen R, Follet A, et al. Evaluating the quality of life of patients with restless legs syndrome. *Clin Ther.* 2004; 26:925-935.

5. Winkelman JW, Finn L, Young T. Prevalence and correlates of restless legs syndrome symptoms in the Wisconsin Sleep Cohort. *Sleep Med.* 2006;7:545-552.

6. Kuzniar TJ, Silber MH. Multiple skeletal injuries resulting from uncontrolled restless legs syndrome. *J Clin Sleep Med.* 2007; 3:60-61.

7. Pearson VE, Allen RP, Dean T, Gamaldo CE, Lesage SR, Earley CJ. Cognitive deficits associated with restless legs syndrome (RLS). *Sleep Med.* 2006;7:25-30.

8. Galmaldo CE, Benbrook AR, Allen RP, Oguntimein O, Earley CJ. A further evaluation of the cognitive deficits associated with restless legs syndrome. *Sleep Med.* 2008;9:500-505.

9. Picchietti D, Winkelman JW. Restless legs syndrome, periodic limb movements in sleep, and depression. *Sleep.* 2005;28:891-898.

10. Winkelmann J, Prager M, Lieb R, et al. "Anxietas tibiarum". Depression and anxiety disorders in patients with restless legs syndrome. *J Neurol.* 2005;252:67-71.

11. Breslau N, Roth T, Rosenthal L, Andreski P. Sleep disturbance and psychiatric disorders: a longitudinal epidemiological study of young adults. *Biol Psychiatry.* 1996;39:411-418.

12. Innes KE, Selfe TK, Agarwal P. Restless legs syndrome and conditions associated with metabolic dysregulation, sympathoadrenal dysfunction, and cardiovascular disease risk: a systematic review. *Sleep Med Rev.* 2012;16:309-339.

5

13. Ulfberg J, Nystrom B, Carter N, Edling C. Prevalence of restless legs syndrome among men aged 18 to 64 years: an association with somatic disease and neuropsychiatric symptoms. *Mov Disord.* 2001;16:1159-1163.

14. Winkelman JW, Shahar E, Sharief I, Gottlieb DJ. Association of restless legs syndrome and cardiovascular disease in the Sleep Heart Health Study. *Neurol.* 2008;70:35-42.

15. Li Y, Walters A, Chiuve SE, Rimm EB, Winkelman JW, Gao X. Prospective study of restless legs syndrome and coronary heart disease among women. *Circulation.* 2012;126:1689-1694.

16. Walters AS, Rye DB. Review of the relationship of restless legs syndrome and periodic limb movements in sleep to hypertension, heart disease, and stroke. *Sleep.* 2009;32:589-597.

6

Diagnosis and Evaluation

Diagnosis of RLS proceeds along the lines suggested in *Chapter 2*: taking the history from the patient to determine if the five diagnostic features of RLS are present and probing to make sure that the patient is not describing a mimic. **Table 6.1** outlines the steps to complete the initial evaluation. A recent review covers many of the diagnostic and assessment instruments.[1]

Diagnostic Instruments

A number of diagnostic instruments have been developed for RLS. For screening purposes, a single question has proved to be sensitive and useful; it identifies majority of all individuals with RLS of any degree.[2,3] The question is: *When you try to relax in the evening or sleep at night, do you ever have unpleasant, restless feelings in your legs that can be relieved by walking or movement?*

However, a single question cannot accurately diagnose RLS as it lacks specificity. Depending on the setting, only 25% to 66% of those who answer "yes" to this question will be found to have RLS. A positive response to this screening question must be followed by a series of more specific diagnostic questions. Two sets of questions are shown in **Table 6.2** and **Table 6.3** that match the 2002 NIH Diagnostic Criteria for RLS and are more specific than the single question screener. These questions based on previous "four diagnostic criteria," however, have generally been used for epidemiologic studies only. Hening and colleagues found that these questions also lack specificity as they are unable to exclude confounding conditions (aka, "mimics").[4]

For a more definitive diagnosis, the Hopkins Telephone Diagnostic Interview (HTDI) is a structured

TABLE 6.1 — Initial Work-Up of RLS

History
- To elucidate symptoms and exclude mimics
- Information on sleep and nighttime motor activity from patient and bed partner or observer
- Review of systems to determine possible causes of

Physical
- Primarily to find possible mimic disorders, causes of RLS, or comorbid conditions that might shape therapy
- Close examination of legs and associated neurologic exam most important

Laboratory
- Blood tests for iron status should be done (ferritin, TIBC, % saturation)
- Screen for anemia, diabetes, and renal failure
- Other blood tests only on clinical suspicion
- Electrodiagnostic tests only if there is suspicion of nerve damage
- Polysomnography (sleep study) not routinely indicated, but may be needed if diagnosis is difficult or an additional sleep disorder suspected
- Suggested immobilization tests or actigraphic monitoring of leg activity may be useful adjuncts

set of questions to both diagnose RLS and determine certain elements of its course. The interview comprises five questions which cover the four essential criteria and a number of other questions about the clinical status of those diagnosed and supplementary questions that attempt to enhance differential diagnosis. The telephone-based version of HTDI has been validated and found to be quite accurate but requires specific training for optimal use.[5,6] In-person administration of HTDI, especially accompanied by a full neurologic examination by a physician, is likely to be even more specific and sensitive than the telephone-based administration.

Another well-validated structured assessment method is the RLS Diagnostic Index (RLS-DI) that consists of 10 items that cover nearly all essential and supportive features of the 2002 NIH diagnostic criteria

TABLE 6.2 — Epidemiologic Questionnaire for RLS

Answers to the first three questions should be either YES or NO:

1. Do you have unpleasant sensations (culturally specific descriptor examples) in your legs combined with an urge or need to move your legs?
2. Do these feelings/symptoms occur mainly or only at rest and do they improve with movement?
3. Are these feelings/symptoms worse in the evening or night than in the morning?
4. How often do these feelings/symptoms occur?
   A. <Once/year
   B. At least once a year but <once/month
   C. Once a month
   D. 2 to 4 times/month
   E. 2 to 3 times/week
   F. 4 to 5 times/week
   G. 6 to 7 times/week

Diagnosis of RLS requires a YES answer to the first three questions.

Berger K, et al. *J Neurol*. 2002;249:1195-1199; Allen RP, et al. *Sleep Med*. 2003;4:101-119.

and two associated features: sleep disturbances and findings of a neurologic assessment. A total score is determined from the answers to the items that represents a measure of probability or certainly of RLS diagnosis. High sensitivity (93%) and specificity (99%) were reported in comparison with the consensus "true" diagnosis of two independent RLS experts.[7]

Sleep Diaries

Sleep diaries can be used to chart the occurrence of RLS symptoms and the time of sleep (**Figure 6.1**). They can cover different time periods, but plotting hourly for 5 days to 2 weeks can reveal the frequency and time of day of symptoms, as well as their impact on sleep. This can be helpful in determining the timing of medication

TABLE 6.3 — Validated Patient-Completed Questionnaire

1. Do you have, or have you had, recurrent uncomfortable feelings or sensations in your legs while you are sitting or lying down?
   - ❏ Yes
   - ❏ No

2. Do you have, or have you had, a feeling of a recurrent need or urge to move your leg while you were sitting or lying down?
   - ❏ Yes
   - ❏ No

If you answered YES to either question, continue with Question 3; otherwise STOP.

3. Are these feelings *always* due to muscle cramps?
   - ❏ Yes
   - ❏ No, they are *not always* due to cramps
   - ❏ Don't know

NOTE: If you answered NO or DON'T KNOW to Question 3, then answer the rest of the questions ONLY for those feelings that are NOT muscle cramps.

4. Are you more likely to have these feelings when you are resting (either sitting or lying down) or when you are physically active?
   - ❏ Resting
   - ❏ Active

5. If you get up and move around when you have these feelings, do these feelings get any better while you actually keep moving?
   - ❏ Yes
   - ❏ No
   - ❏ Don't know

6. Which times of day are these feelings in your legs most likely to occur? *(Please mark all that apply, ie, one or more than one)*

□ Morning ☐ Evening
☐ Mid-day ☐ Night
☐ Afternoon ☐ About equal at all times

---

7. When you actually experience the feelings in your legs, how *distressing* are they?

☐ Not at all distressing
☐ A little bit distressing
☐ Moderately distressing
☐ Extremely distressing

---

8. In the past 12 months, how often did you experience these feelings in your legs? *(Please mark only one answer)*

☐ Every day ☐ 2 days/month
☐ 4-6 days/week ☐ 1 day/month
☐ 2-3 days/week ☐ <1 day/month
☐ 1 day/week ☐ Never

---

9. Approximately how old were you when you first noticed these feelings in your legs? *(Please write age)*

_____ Years of age

Diagnosis depends on questions 1 through 6. Questions 7 through 9 provide a basic characterization of the disorder. To have definite RLS, you must answer YES to Questions 1 and 2, YES or Don't Know to 3, Resting to 4, YES to 5, and 6 should include evening and night, although in very severe cases other times may be mentioned. Persons who answer NO to Question 1, but answer the remainder of the questions consistent with RLS may be diagnosed as probable RLS.

Nichols DA, et al. *Sleep.* 2003;36(suppl):A346.

FIGURE 6.1 — Example of a Sleep Diary in a Patient With Severe RLS

		Mid-day/Noon		Afternoon				Evening						Midnight						Morning						
DATE	DAY	12-1	1-2	2-3	3-4	4-5	5-6	6-7	7	8	9	10	11	12-1	1-2	2-3	3-4	4-5	5-6	6-7	7	8	9	10	11	
	Monday	r	r	R	R	R	R	R	R	R	R	R	V	R	R	R	R	r↓	r✶	←•	r	r	r	r	r	Tuesday
	Tuesday	•	•	•	•	r	r	R	R	R	R	R	V/R	R	R	R	R	r→	r→	↑	•	•	•	•	•	Wednesday
1/26/00	Wednesday	•	•	•	•	•	•	r	•	•	r	R V/R	R	R↓	R↓	R	R	←R	↑	•	•	•	•	•	•	Thursday
1/27/00	Thursday	•	•	•	r→	r	•	r	r	r	R	R V½	V½	R↓	r R	r R	←R	R	•	←•	•	•	•	•	•	Friday
1/28/00	Friday	•	•	•	•	r	r	•	r	•	R	r	r	R	R	r→	↓	↓		→	•	•	•	•	•	Saturday
1/29/00	Saturday	•	•	•	r	•	r	•	•	•	•	r	r	R	R	r	↓	↓	↓	↓	←•	•	•	•	•	Sunday
1/30/00	Sunday	•	•	•	•	•	•	•	•	•	•	•	r	r	r	↓	↓	↓	←	r	•	•	•			Monday
1/31/00	Monday			Dosing with iron										R	R	→	↓	→	•	•						Tuesday

Symptoms are marked for each hour of the day; R = restless legs during the hour; small r for mild or little amount of RLS; capital R for disturbing amount). The patient also marks when going to bed (↓) and when rising (↑). Time spent actually asleep is filled in; part way into a block indicates part way into the hour. A letter code indicates any sleep-related medication taken and in what hour.

Sample courtesy of the RLS Center, Johns Hopkins Bayview Medical Center, Baltimore, MD.

doses and ascertaining how well a treatment is working. Electronic diaries are available that can be combined with actigraphy, although these are usually reserved for basic research or therapeutic studies.

The Medical Outcome Scales for Sleep (MOS) can also provide a subjective assessment for the period of sleep and sleep satisfaction.[8,9] A similar instrument, the Pittsburgh Sleep Quality Index, can also be used to examine aspects of sleep quality.[10,11]

Rating Scales for RLS

The Johns Hopkins Rating Scale (**Table 6.4**)[12] judges severity by the time of symptom onset. Because it is designed to differentiate those with daily or near-daily symptoms, it is less useful for evaluating the severity of milder cases of RLS.

TABLE 6.4 — Johns Hopkins Restless Legs Syndrome Scale (JHRLSS)

No restless legs syndrome (RLS)	0
Less than almost daily	0.5
Symptoms at bedtime or during sleep	1
Symptoms begin after 18:00 but before bedtime	2
Symptoms begin before 18:00	3
Symptoms begin before noon	4

Before applying, a diagnosis of RLS must be made and the rating applied strictly to RLS symptoms.

Allen RP, et al. *Sleep Med*. 2001;2:239-242.

The International RLS Study group rating scale (**Appendix A**) has been one of the most commonly used primary outcome measures in RLS therapeutic clinical trials. It has been validated and has been found to have excellent psychometric properties.[13-16] This scale measures both the symptoms of RLS and also the impact on sleep, daytime function, mood, and daily activities. It can be seen as having two main factors: symptoms and impact,[17] with sleep bridging the two.[16,18]

The CGI[19] is a summary measure that is used by the treating clinician to assess the condition of the patient (**Table 6.5**). It can be used as a quick way of measuring RLS, although it is a flexible tool that can be applied to many disorders. It has also been used as an important outcome measure in many therapeutic trials. There is also a patient variant of the measure, which is then called a Patient Global Impression, and follows the same form but has the rating assigned by the patient, rather than the clinician.

TABLE 6.5 — Clinical Global Impression (CGI)

CGI—Severity of Illness (CGI-S)
- 7-point scale from 1 = not at all ill through 7 = severely ill

CGI—Improvement or Change (CGI-I)
- 7-point scale ranging from –3 = very much improved through 0 = unchanged to 3 = very much worse

CGI—Therapeutic Improvement
- 4-point scale from 1 = very good (much or very much improved) to 4 = unchanged or worse

CGI—Tolerability (adverse events)
- 4-point scale from 1 = no adverse events to 4 = adverse events outweigh benefits

The first two scales, CGI-S and CGI-I, are the ones most used in clinical trials. The Patient Global Impression follows the same format and scoring, but the judgment is made by the patient rather than the clinician or investigator.

The RLS-6 Scales (**Table 6.6**) have been used primarily in Europe. These scales ask about the severity of RLS symptoms in different situations and times of day, as well as a global sleep assessment. These are visual analogue scales in which the individual assigns a point along a continuum to the degree of current symptoms in each setting. As to be expected, the scales asking about nighttime and sleep are the most heavily endorsed by patients as more bothersome.

Another related scale is the Augmentation Severity Rating Scale (ASRS; **Appendix A**, **Figure A.1**) that

TABLE 6.6 — RLS-6 Scales

Each scale is a visual analogue scale in which the patient or subject places a mark at the point on a (usually) 10-cm line that is marked into 10 segments. The score is determined by measurement of the mark with distance converted into an 11-point 0-to-10 score, where 0 indicates no relevant symptoms/complaints and 10 is the most severe.

1. RLS symptoms at bedtime

2. RLS symptoms during the night

3. RLS symptoms at rest during the daytime

4. RLS symptoms when active during the daytime

5. Satisfaction with sleep

6. Daytime fatigue and tiredness

The first two items tend to show the greatest symptoms, while the fourth item is usually rated very low.

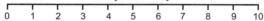

provides a quantitative measure of the severity of augmentation. Primarily developed for the purpose of assessing augmentation—a main complication during long-term dopaminergic treatment associated with worsening of RLS symptoms—this three-item rating scale is to be assessed at baseline and then administered prospectively with treatment. Reliability and validity of ASRS has been established and ASRS has become a vital assessment instrument in RLS clinical trials.[20]

Quality of Life

Very important sequelae of RLS include an impaired quality of life (QOL). Some studies of RLS have used the SF-36, a standard, general measure of QOL in eight physical and psychological domains,[21] to assess quality of life in RLS patients. It has been shown that QOL is impaired in RLS and that the QOL decreases with greater severity of RLS (**Figure 6.2**).[22-]

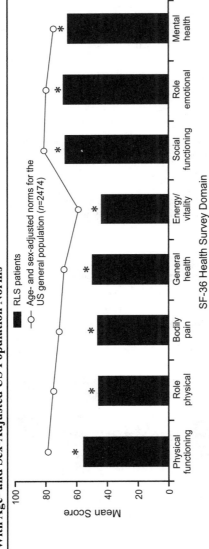

FIGURE 6.2 — Short-Form 36 Health Survey Scores of Patients With RLS With Age- and Sex-Adjusted US Population Norms

Asterisks indicate that the scores of the RLS-sufferer group were significantly below the norms for all eight dimensions.

Allen RP, et al. *Arch Intern Med.* 2005;165:1286-1292.

[24] This decrease in those with significant RLS (twice or greater per week and bothersome symptoms) is comparable to chronic medical conditions such as type 2 diabetes. There are now also two RLS-specific QOL scales developed to measure the consequences of RLS symptoms and sleep loss in relation to QOL. The RLS quality of life instrument (RLS-QOL) is factored with four domains (daily function, social function, sleep quality, and emotional well-being) and has been validated and found to have good psychometric qualities.[25] The RLS-QOL provides a single measure of disorder impact and has also been validated.[26]

Physical Examination

As indicated in **Table 6.1**, the major purpose of the physical examination in RLS is to search for causative or comorbid conditions or to make findings to help with the differential diagnosis. Careful attention should be paid to the legs, with evaluation of any lesions, joint abnormalities, venous engorgement, or decreased pulse. The neurologic exam should determine if there is any loss of sensation in the various modalities and check reflexes and muscle strength, primarily to look for polyneuropathy, radiculopathy, or mononeuropathy. Other aspects of the physical exam may also suggest a systemic process that may be important for assessment.

Laboratory Evaluation

The most essential laboratory assessment is to check for iron status, using ferritin (a measure of body iron stores), total binding capacity, and percent saturation. The serum iron level itself is generally not useful. The presence of ferritin <50 mcg/L should trigger considerations of therapeutic iron repletion and levels <30 mcg/L should be followed by a full work-up for iron deficiency. Percent saturation <20% has a similar implication. In patients who develop significant treatment resistance or have a sudden deterioration, a follow-up test may reveal newly developed iron deficiency. It must be remembered, however, that ferritin is also an acute-phase inflammatory reactant, so the measure has a questionable value during any acute illness.

A complete blood count can help identify anemia, which may be associated with iron deficiency. Screening for diabetes (blood glucose or glycosylated hemoglobin) or uremia (BUN, creatinine) may be helpful. Other screening for possible causes, such as B_{12} deficiency or autoimmune factors (eg, suggesting rheumatoid arthritis) has not proved useful[27] and should only be pursued when there is some additional reason to suspect such disorders (ie, history or findings on physical exam).

Electrodiagnostic studies to assess nerve function should also be restricted to those who show clear signs of nerve dysfunction (sensory loss, atrophy, weakness) or have a history of progressive numbness or weakness, either generalized or in a restricted distribution. The relationship of RLS to nerve dysfunction is unclear. Much of the nerve dysfunction in RLS involves small fibers whose integrity is not evaluated by standard nerve conduction tests or electromyography.[28-30] In any case, RLS treatment is not much altered by these findings, although there may be some greater preference for using an anticonvulsant such as gabapentin.[30,31]

The PSG or sleep study is a standard means of assessing sleep (**Table 6.7**). It measures the length and depth of sleep, the time it takes to get to sleep, and the number of arousals and awakenings. Respiration is measured to determine if there are any sleep-related respiratory disorders. In most studies, leg muscle activity is measured with an EMG to record motor activity, including PLM. Typical abnormal findings from RLS are indicated in **Table 6.8**. These, however, are not considered diagnostic; the American Academy of Sleep Medicine standards indicate that a PSG is not necessary for the routine diagnosis of RLS.[32] Those situations in which a PSG might be useful in RLS include cases of

TABLE 6.7 — The Polysomnogram (Sleep Study)

State Measurement—

These can provide measures of latency to sleep onset and quantity of sleep, different sleep stages (REM and NREM), stage shifts, wakenings, arousals:

- EEG recording: usually at least two leads, one central (C3-A2) and one occipital (O2-A1)
- Eye movement recording: electro-oculogram to measure movement in eyes
- Chin EMG to measure brachial muscle tone

Respiratory Measurement—

This can detect breathing effort and any cessations of breathing (apnea) or diminution (hypopnea). Nasal cannula can determine excess breathing effort (upper airway resistance syndrome):

- Belts to record thoracic and abdominal breathing effort
- Thermistor to record nasal and buccal airflow or nasal cannula to measure pressure
- Oximeter to measure oxygen saturation

Movement Activity—

These can record PLM; in conjunction with mentalis EMG and artifacts on EEG traces, these can indicate generalized movement:

- Bilateral anterior tibialis EMG

Cardiac Measurement

- EKG

Special studies looking for movement disorders or epilepsy may require additional EEG and/or EMG channels.

---

uncertain diagnosis, cases where another sleep disorder is suspected, and cases where treatment with the usual RLS medications has not been helpful.

The SIT (**Table 2.3**) can be combined with the PSG to gain a clearer picture of RLS. The SIT is performed immediately before the PSG begins, later in the evening (eg, 22:00), since sensory discomfort increases as the time advances towards midnight (**Figure 6.3**). As time goes on, this test may prove to be more important in assessing therapies, especially those aimed at intermittent symptoms.

TABLE 6.8 — Typical RLS Findings on a Sleep Study

Sleep States
- Prolonged sleep latency (wake before sleep onset)
- Increased arousals and awakenings
- Increased wake during the night (wake after sleep onset)
- Increased light sleep (non–rapid eye movement stage 1)

Respiratory
- Nothing typical, but RLS can be associated with sleep related breathing disorders[1]

Movement Activity
- Increased periodic limb movements in sleep (usually >5/hour, typically >15/hour)
- Increased periodic limb movements in wake
- Restlessness recorded as generalized movements (epochs scored as movement time)

Cardiac
- Nothing typical, but RLS can be associated with cardiac disorders that may be reflected in abnormal rhythms

[1]Lakshminarayanan S, et al. *Mov Disord.* 2005;20:502-503.

Actigraphy, as discussed in *Chapter 2*, can be used to gain a more extended picture of sleep continuity and PLM than the PSG. Actigraphic measurement of activity, either over 24 hours or at night, can provide useful information for shaping treatment. Actigraphy can also be combined with sleep diaries, either paper or electronic, to associate symptom level with motor activity and sleep.

FIGURE 6.3 — Sensory Discomfort During Suggested Immobilization Test

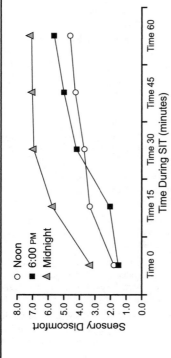

This presents data from 11 subjects who had SITs performed at 3-hour intervals with intervening activity. The SITs lasted 60 minutes and sensory discomfort from RLS was rated at the beginning of the SIT and every 15 minutes thereafter. Discomfort was rated on a visual analogue scale of 10 cm running from 0 (no symptoms) to 10 (most severe symptoms possible).

Data reported is based on Hening WA, et al. *Sleep.* 1999;22:901-912.

REFERENCES

1. Kohnen R, Allen RP, Benes H, et al. Assessment of restless legs syndrome. Methodological approaches for use in practice and clinical trials. *Mov Disord.* 2007;22:S485-S494.

2. Ferri R, Lanuzza B, Cosentino FH, et al. A single question for the rapid screening of restless legs syndrome in the neurological clinical practice. *Eur J Neurol.* 2007;14(9):1016-1021.

3. Hening WA, Sharon D, Abraham M, et al. Validation of a single question screener question for the Restless Legs Syndrome. *Mov Disord.* 2006;21(suppl):S443. Abstract.

4. Hening WA, Allen RP, Washburn M, Lesage SR, Earley CJ. The our diagnostic criteria for Restless legs Syndrome are unable to exclude confounding conditions ("mimics"). 2009;10:976-981.

5. Hening W, Washburn M, Allen R, Lesage S, Earley C. Validation of the Hopkins telephone diagnostic interview for the restless legs syndrome. *Sleep Med.* 2008;9:283-289.

6. Hening WA, Allen RP, Thanner S, et al. The Johns Hopkins telephone diagnostic interview for the restless legs syndrome: preliminary investigation for validation in a multi-center patient and control population. *Sleep Med.* 2003;4:137-141.

7. Benes H, Kohnen R. Validation of an algorithm for diagnosis of restless legs syndrome: the restless legs syndrome-diagnostic index (RLS-DI). *Sleep Med.* 2009;10:515-523.

8. Stewart AL, Hays RD, Ware JE Jr. The MOS short-form general health survey. Reliability and validity in a patient population. *Med Care.* 1988;26:724-735.

9. Cunningham WE, Hays RD, Burton TM, Kington RS. Health status measurement performance and health status differences by age, ethnicity, and gender: assessment in the medical outcomes study. *J Health Care Poor Underserved.* 2000;11:58-76.

10. Cole JC, Motivala SJ, Buysse DJ, Oxman MN, Levin MJ, Irwin MR. Validation of a 3-factor scoring model for the Pittsburgh sleep quality index in older adults. *Sleep.* 2006;29:112-116.

11. Backhaus J, Junghanns K, Broocks A, Riemann D, Hohagen F. Test-retest reliability and validity of the Pittsburgh Sleep Quality Index in primary insomnia. *J Psychosom Res.* 2002;53:737-740.

12. Allen RP, Earley CJ. Validation of the Johns Hopkins restless legs severity scale. *Sleep Med.* 2001;2:239-242.

13. Walters AS, LeBrocq C, Dhar A, et al; International Restless Legs Syndrome Study Group. Validation of the International Restless Legs Syndrome Study Group rating scale for restless legs syndrome. *Sleep Med.* 2003;4:121-132.

14. Garcia-Borreguero D, Larrosa O, de la Llave Y, Granizo JJ, Allen R. Correlation between rating scales and sleep laboratory measurements in restless legs syndrome. *Sleep Med.* 2004;5:561-565.

15. Wunderlich GR, Evans KR, Sills T, et al. An item response analysis of the international restless legs syndrome study group rating scale for restless legs syndrome. *Sleep Med.* 2005;6:131-139.

16. Abetz L, Arbuckle R, Allen RP, et al. The reliability, validity and responsiveness of the International Restless Legs Syndrome Study Group rating scale and subscales in a clinical-trial setting. *Sleep Med.* 2006;7:340-349.

17. Allen RP, Kushida CA, Atkinson MJ; RLS QoL Consortium. Factor analysis of the International Restless Legs Syndrome Study Group's scale for restless legs severity. *Sleep Med.* 2003; 4:133-135.

18. Kushida CA, Allen RP, Atkinson MJ. Modeling the causal relationships between symptoms associated with restless legs syndrome and the patient-reported impact of RLS. *Sleep Med.* 2004;5:485-488.

19. National Institute of Mental Health, CGI. Clinical global impressions. In: Guy W, ed. *ECDEU Assessment Manual for Psychopharmacology*. Rockville, MD: National Institute of Mental Health; 1976:218-222.

20. Garcia-Borreguero D, Kohnen R, Hogl B, et al. Validation of the Augmentation Severity Rating Scale (ASRS): a multicentric, prospective study with levodopa on restless legs syndrome. *Sleep Med.* 2007;8:455-463.

21. Ware JE. SF-36 *Health Survey—Manual and Interpretation Guide*. Boston, MA: Massachusetts Health Institute, New England Medical Center; 1993.

22. Allen RP, Walters AS, Montplaisir J, et al. Restless legs syndrome prevalence and impact: REST general population study. *Arch Intern Med.* 2005;165:1286-1292.

23. Kushida C, Martin M, Nikam P, et al. Burden of restless legs syndrome on health-related quality of life. *Qual Life Res.* 2007; 16:617-624.

6

24. Abetz L, Allen R, Follet A, et al. Evaluating the quality of life of patients with restless legs syndrome. *Clin Ther*. 2004; 26:925-935.

25. Atkinson MJ, Allen RP, DuChane J, Murray C, Kushida C, Roth T; RLS Quality of Life Consortium. Validation of the Restless Legs Syndrome Quality of Life Instrument (RLS-QLI): findings of a consortium of national experts and the RLS Foundation. *Qual Life Res*. 2004;13:679-693.

26. Abetz L, Arbuckle R, Allen RP, Mavraki E, Kirsch J. The reliability, validity and responsiveness of the Restless Legs Syndrome Quality of Life questionnaire (RLSQoL) in a trial population. *Health Qual Life Outcomes*. 2005;3:79.

27. Ondo W, Tan EK, Mansoor J. Rheumatologic serologies in secondary restless legs syndrome. *Mov Disord*. 2000;15:321-323.

28. Polydefkis M, Allen RP, Hauer P, Earley CJ, Griffin JW, McArthur JC. Subclinical sensory neuropathy in late-onset restless legs syndrome. *Neurology*. 2000;55:1115-1121.

29. Gemignani F, Brindani F, Negrotti A, Vitetta F, Alfieri S, Marbini A. Restless legs syndrome and polyneuropathy. *Mov Disord*. 2006;21:1254-1257.

30. Gemignani F, Brindani F, Vitetta F, Marbini A, Calzetti S. Restless legs syndrome in diabetic neuropathy: a frequent manifestation of small fiber neuropathy. *J Peripher Nerv Syst*. 2007;12:50-53.

31. Garcia-Borreguero D, Larrosa O, de la Llave Y, Verger K, Masramon X, Hernandez G. Treatment of restless legs syndrome with gabapentin: a double-blind, cross-over study. *Neurology*. 2002;59:1573-1579.

32. Kushida CA, Littner MR, Morgenthaler T, et al. Practice parameters for the indications for polysomnography and related procedures: an update for 2005. *Sleep*. 2005;28:499-521.

7 Management

A spectrum of treatment options are available to address the wide range in severity and frequency of RLS symptoms. This chapter will outline a logical approach for initiating and individualizing treatment for RLS patients.[1] The general guide to treatment decisions is outlined in **Table 7.1**.

Tailoring Treatment to Symptoms

■ **When to Treat**?

When to treat is a common question that arises with any condition that causes discomfort or pain. When symptoms are frequent and severe, the decision is quite simple: Effective therapy should be instituted promptly. However, this decision is not as straightforward with less severe cases.

Mild and infrequent RLS symptoms often do not need to be treated. However, individuals can differ in their response to symptoms, and even mild and infrequent symptoms may result in significant disability for some.

Decisions on how to treat RLS depend on the degree of discomfort and lifestyle disturbance a particular patient experiences. Most people who experience mild RLS symptoms on an infrequent basis do not need drug therapy. However, if they have problems when sitting for prolonged periods of time, they may not be able attend school, work at sedentary jobs, go to the movies or the theater, or travel by airplane. Although these symptoms may often have no impact on the majority of their life, they may preclude their ability to participate in or enjoy sedentary activities. These restrictions, especially if they impact the ability to work or school, often require treatment.

TABLE 7.1 — General Guide to Treatment Decisions in Patients With RLS

When to Treat?
- Is RLS clinically significant? Frequent and severe enough to merit treatment?
- If so, what is the appropriate intervention?
  - Consider lifestyle, nonpharmacologic interventions
  - Frequency of symptoms determines when therapy is needed vs daily treatment
  - Severity of symptoms—how bothersome are symptoms? Do they compromise life activities (social, occupational, or educational) or sleep? Do they affect behavior, mood, or cognition?

Timing of Doses?
- Time or situation of occurrence of symptoms
- Time to onset of drug action
- Consider longer-acting drugs for those with daytime symptoms or daytime symptom breakthrough

Adjustment of Treatment
- Routine follow-up
- Monitor for adverse effects, degree of relief
- Always check iron status: serum iron, TIBC, and serum ferritin
- Be alert to changes in response:
  - Change in patient condition, other treatments, lifestyle changes
  - Consider tolerance, augmentation, and disease progression

Each person with RLS should be assessed for the severity, frequency, and timing of their symptoms. Once these parameters are determined and how much they disturb the person's life, it should be easier to decide whether to initiate treatment.

However, it is often difficult to ascertain whether the RLS symptoms are causing enough disruption to warrant treatment. Symptoms are often present for years or even decades before they come to the attention of a physician and are typically downplayed or even ignored. People with undiagnosed RLS often believe that their symptoms are normal feelings that everyone may experience or are so strange that they do not deserve to be treated. Many patients may not be fully aware of the degree that they have adjusted their lifestyle to avoid suffering from RLS symptoms. They will avoid going to movies, theater, and other sedentary social events (especially in the evenings which may isolate them socially) and may change their schedule to perform sedentary functions early in the day when symptoms are less provoked while engaging in active ones (laundry, exercise) later in the day. Once a diagnosis of RLS is made, the patient should be carefully questioned to determine the true degree of suffering and disability from this disorder.

■ Timing of Symptoms

The timing of RLS symptoms is a key factor in the decision of whether and how to treat. Generally, symptoms tend to peak at bedtime but many may experience symptoms earlier or later on in the day. People whose symptoms occur mainly in the early evening or late afternoon have the option of being more active at these times and may not need any drug treatment.

However, if they need or wish to participate in sedentary activities (school, work, movies, theater, travel) at these times, treatment may be essential. With time, most people know which activities and at which times and durations that their RLS symptoms will be provoked. They can thus take preventive treatment beforehand and completely avoid the emergence of any RLS symptoms.

Symptoms that occur while trying to fall asleep at bedtime tend to be more troublesome. They can easily disrupt the initiation or maintenance of sleep and result in significant insomnia. However, if the symptoms are mild such that they cause only a short delay in falling asleep or getting back to sleep, treatment should not be necessary.

Different drugs should be considered depending upon the time that the symptoms occur. Daytime symptoms are better treated with nonsedating drugs, while sedating drugs may be more appropriate for bedtime RLS symptoms. Drugs that onset quickly are better suited for unexpected symptoms (especially at bedtime) while slower-acting drugs can be prescribed for anticipated problems (eg, movies or airplane trips).

Patient with more severe RLS will often have symptoms that occur earlier in the day usually starting in the afternoon or even upon awakening. Those patients may benefit from multiple doses of short-acting medications (which may give them the option of omitting doses when more active) or from a longer-acting drug that can provide continuous relief with more convenient dosing. As noted, patients may often not be aware of their lifestyle modifications and may unconsciously avoid sedentary situations due to fear of breakthrough RLS symptoms. Exploring these issues can prove helpful since treatment with a longer-acting medication that may provide a higher quality of life with less worry about manipulating their lifestyles or medications.

■ Frequency and Severity of Symptoms

As previously discussed, mild and infrequent RLS symptoms usually do not need to be treated with medication. These symptoms typically can be managed with nonpharmacologic therapy (see *Chapter 8*).

However, RLS symptoms that are very severe but occur infrequently or less-severe RLS symptoms that occur more frequently may require treatment with drugs. Since it is often hard to determine the severity of RLS symptoms (although several rating scales exist), it may be easier to estimate the severity by the effect the symptoms have on the person's life. Treatment should be considered for any symptoms that are intense enough to be disruptive and affect the person's quality of life.

When symptoms are less severe, treatment may be determined by their frequency. Chronic persistent symptoms that occur daily generally require drug therapy. However, symptoms occurring two to four times per week or more (especially if they cause significant insomnia or disruption of other sedentary activities) may also require daily treatment. It is important to discuss these issues with the patient and determine the impact of their symptoms before prescribing medication. The classification of RLS patients discussed below and the "Specifiers for Clinical Significance for RLS" in the IRLSSG diagnostic criteria (see *Chapter 2*) were designed to highlight the complex interaction of frequency and severity of symptoms.

■ **Comorbid and Other Underlying Conditions**

When initiating therapy, the patient's other medical problems should be taken into consideration. Patients with depression should avoid RLS drugs ($\alpha2\delta$ ligand) that could potentially worsen depressive symptoms, but patients with anxiety may benefit from these drugs. Comorbid pain syndromes (especially painful neuropathy which is often associated with RLS) may be helped by $\alpha2\delta$ ligands or even opioids. As noted, RLS patients with insomnia may benefit from sedating RLS drugs, such as the $\alpha2\delta$ ligands.

The metabolism of the drug should be considered and either adjusted or avoided for those with hepatic or renal impairment. Drugs that may cause weight gain should be used with caution in obese patients and drugs that tend to worsen sleep apnea should also been used with caution while monitoring for development or exacerbation of sleep disordered breathing that may require an appropriate treatment response. Patients with a history of substance abuse may not be appropriate candidates for opioid therapy. Patients who are on multiple drugs that undergo hepatic metabolism may do better with drugs that are excreted by the kidneys (eg, $\alpha2\delta$ ligands). Pregnant RLS patient should avoid Category C drugs (dopamine agonists, $\alpha2\delta$ ligands) as they pose a significant risk to the fetus.

Iron deficiency (with or without anemia) should be ruled out as it is fairly common in RLS patients and iron-supplement treatment may improve RLS symptoms. Even with normal CBC, serum iron, and

TIBC levels, serum ferritin levels (representing iron stores) may be low and treating patients with levels <50-75 mcg/L[1] (rather than the usual lab normal range of >10-20 mcg/L) may be beneficial. Iron status should be checked initially, once a year on a follow-up visit, or when an unexplained exacerbation occurs.

■ Follow the Patient

Although many patients remain stable for years after starting treatment, it is quite common for RLS to worsen gradually over years to decades. Some patients have wide fluctuations in their symptoms, which may be due to other medications, hormonal changes, concomitant disease, work situation, augmentation (see *Chapter 9*), loss of drug efficacy, or other reasons that may not always be apparent. It is therefore essential to follow the patient with periodic recheck visits to reassess their symptoms and medication needs.

Medication regimens should be flexible enough to cover the fluctuations that are common among RLS sufferers. Although patients can often prevent RLS symptoms by taking their medication in a timely fashion, this is not always the case. It is a good idea to add a fast-acting medication for those occasions when symptoms present unexpectedly or occur due to lack of adherence to the medication schedule.

Classification of RLS Patients

There are several ways in which RLS patients may be categorized to help guide treatment protocols. One of the more practical classifications for managing people with RLS was developed by a group of RLS specialists to create an algorithm for guiding the treatment of the disorder.[2] Below is this classification with some additional modifications based on updated guidelines from the IRLSSG,[3] which will be used in subsequent chapters to discuss the management of RLS. It is outlined in **Table 7.2**.

TABLE 7.2 — Classification of RLS Patients

Intermittent RLS Patients
- Symptoms when not treated would occur on average <2 per week for the past year with at least five lifetime events
- Usually milder symptoms compared with chronic persistent patients
- Symptoms often situational and/or predictable

Chronic Persistent/Daily RLS Patients
- Symptoms when not treated would occur on average at least twice a week for the past year but usually more frequent and often daily
- Symptoms are typically more severe and tend to impact social, occupational, or educational aspects of life

Refractory RLS Patients
- Failure of available first-line therapy (at least one adequate trial of a first-line approved dopamine agonist and if available, an $\alpha 2\delta$ ligand)
- Generally indicates that therapeutic effect has diminished; may be due to tolerance, progression, and/or augmentation
- Several strategies available for dealing with these patients

It should be noted that all of the FDA-approved drugs are recommended for treating moderate to severe RLS. The designation of moderate to severe is based on the IRLS (International RLSSG) scores of ≥ 15 (see *Appendix A*). The IRLS score is determined by adding the results of 10 questions (rated from 0-4) for a maximum of 40 points. Although all the studies to obtain FDA approval were performed on patients with scores of ≥ 15, moderate RLS is defined as an IRLS score of 11-20 and those patients can be considered for treatment with the FDA approved drugs. Since the IRLS is based on questions that span frequency, severity, and impact of symptoms, the IRLS scores may not fall in any of the three categories defined below that are based on the frequency or lack of response to approved drugs. It is likely that the majority of the patients with moderate to severe RLS will fall into the latter of the three categories below but there may be many exceptions.

■ Intermittent RLS

Intermittent RLS is defined as symptoms when not treated would occur on average <2/week for the past year with at least five lifetime events. These patients are typically easier to manage, as their symptoms tend to be milder and respond more readily to therapy.

Some people with intermittent RLS may experience more intense symptoms, but most in this group will complain of these more intense RLS problems only occasionally (airplane flights, long movies, or meetings). With time (often years to decades), many in this category may progress to more frequent or daily RLS symptoms.

■ Chronic-Persistent/Daily RLS

Chronic-persistent/daily RLS is defined by symptoms when not treated would occur on average at least twice a week for the past year. Although this is a diverse group based on frequency, most tend to have symptoms on a daily basis. Typically, this group is more likely to have moderate to severe symptoms. They are usually more difficult to treat than patients with intermittent RLS and may require higher doses of medication or even combinations of drugs to relieve their symptoms.

■ Refractory RLS

Refractory RLS is defined as chronic-persistent/ daily RLS that has failed available first-line therapy (at least one adequate trial of a first-line, approved dopamine agonist and also if available, an $\alpha2\delta$ ligand) with one or more of the following outcomes:

- Inadequate initial response despite adequate doses
- Response that has become inadequate with time, despite increasing doses
- Intolerable adverse effects

- Augmentation that is not controllable with additional earlier doses of the drug while staying within the approved dose range for a drug

This group tends to be the most difficult to manage. Luckily, they comprise a minority of RLS patients who present to most doctors. However, due to the increased recognition of RLS that has resulted in more patients being treated during the past decade, there has been a steady increase in refractory RLS patients. These patients comprise the majority of patients seen by RLS specialists. Discussion of how to manage and assess these patients is presented in *Chapter 9* and *Chapter 10*.

REFERENCES

1. Wang J, O'Reilly B, Venkataraman R, Mysliwiec V, Mysliwiec A. Efficacy of oral iron in patients with restless legs syndrome and a low-normal ferritin: A randomized, double-blind, placebo-controlled study. *Sleep Med.* 2009;10(9):973-975.

2. Silber MH, Ehrenberg BL, Allen RP, et al; Medical Advisory Board of the Restless Legs Syndrome Foundation. An algorithm for the management of restless legs syndrome. *Mayo Clin Proc.* 2004;79(7):916-922.

3. 2011 Revised IRLSSG Diagnostic Criteria for RLS; Specifiers for Clinical Course of RLS. International Resless Legs Syndrome Study Group Web site. http://irlssg.org/diagnostic-criteria. Accessed March 13, 2013.

8

Nonpharmacologic Management/Lifestyle Modifications

All RLS patients may benefit from the nonpharmacologic management. **Table 8.1** is a listing of nonpharmacologic approaches and resources that should be considered for every RLS patient, regardless of severity or frequency. Many of these approaches will be therapeutic for most people with RLS but others may benefit from only a select few.

Physicians should be familiar with these nonpharmacologic measures since they may provide great relief without risking pharmacologic side effects. Some patients may actually avoid the need for any drugs while others may significantly decrease the amount of medication needed. Therefore, physicians should share this list of nonpharmacologic measures with each patient so that they can discover the ones that may help them. To treat this disorder properly, the doctor and patient must work together as a team, especially with this nonpharmacologic approach to the disorder.

Although some of the treatments described in this chapter are either well documented or studied in the medical literature, many others are not. These therapies are often difficult to test in a scientific manner. Therefore, much of the following information is based on anecdotal evidence gathered from those suffering from RLS and experts in the field.

Even though most physicians favor managing RLS with medication, most patients prefer the nonpharmacologic approach. Whether or not the doctor suggests these therapies, the majority of people with RLS seek them out anyway. Thus it is beneficial to work with the patient and guide them to the safer and more effective nondrug treatments.

TABLE 8.1 — Nonpharmacologic Management of RLS

- Avoid provocative substances:
  - Coffee, alcohol, tobacco
  - Medications:
    - Neuroleptics
    - Antidepressants
    - Antihistamines
    - Antinausea/antiemetics
    - Other dopamine blockers
    - Sedative hypnotics
- Consider RLS-friendly alternatives
- Sleep hygiene:
  - Avoid sleep deprivation
  - Regular hours of sleep
  - Optimize bedroom for sleep
  - Prepare for sleep with relaxing/symptom-reducing activities
- Exercise and physical conditioning
- Alerting activities
- Counterstimulation
- Alternative medical treatments
- Patient organizations and support groups

Avoiding Provocative Substances

As noted, physicians should be familiar with the substances and especially medications that worsen RLS, as these have the potential to become the cause of exacerbating symptoms. When symptoms worsen inexplicitly, physicians should review all new prescription medications and especially OTC drugs as patients often forget to mention them.

■ Dietary and Nutritional Considerations

Despite the fact that there are few, if any, credible studies investigating the role of diet and nutrition on RLS, this is one of the more common measures employed by people with the disorder and often mentioned in review papers.[1] Those suffering from RLS often report that decreasing carbohydrates or gluten may be helpful. Many report that some dairy products such as ice cream tend to trigger RLS.

There is some literature examining the relationship of caffeine, alcohol, and tobacco and RLS. Although these links have not been firmly established, it is reasonable to suggest that people suffering from RLS abstain from these substances to determine if it improves their symptoms. These substances are further discussed below.

Caffeine

There is an early report[2] in 1978 that discussed 10 patients who had complete relief by withdrawing from caffeine-containing beverages, food, medications, and other xanthine-containing products. Most of the patients got rapid relief from their RLS symptoms within the first few days of abstinence. Two of the patients had a return of symptoms upon the resumption of caffeine products.

One study looking at the risk factors of RLS in depressed or anxious patients maintained on tricyclic and serotonin reuptake inhibiting antidepressants found that the regular use of nonopioid analgesics (frequently combined with caffeine) appeared to be the major risk factor for RLS rather than their use of antidepressants.[3]

Clearly, there is no adequate evidence to claim that caffeine exacerbates RLS at the moment. Furthermore, as caffeine is a stimulating substance that increases dopamine release, theoretically, it should decrease the propensity for RLS rather than increase it. Nevertheless, it is prudent to advise people with RLS to determine whether avoiding caffeine is beneficial. This may be difficult due to the pervasiveness of this substance in foods and medications.

Alcohol

Despite alcohol being one of the more commonly used hypnotics, it can cause disturbed sleep. Even a single low dose may result in increased sleep fragmentation and number of awakenings in non–alcohol-dependent adults.[4] Alcohol intake at bedtime shortens the time to onset of sleep but increases wakefulness in the second half of the night,[5] which may then be further exacerbated by the presence of RLS symptoms.

Although no evidence exists to date in the medical literature validating that alcohol exacerbates RLS, this is a common complaint among those with the disorder. It is possible that the sedation created by consuming alcohol may worsen RLS. However, one epidemiologic study using telephone interviews in 1803 Kentucky adults found that RLS was associated with low alcohol consumption.[6]

Tobacco

The association of cigarette smoking and RLS is difficult to discern. There had been a case report of a 70-year-old female smoker with lung disease whose severe and refractory RLS symptoms remitted within 1 month after smoking cessation.[7] However, no association between RLS and smoking was found in a 1997 Canadian epidemiologic survey based on 2019 adults who were asked about RLS symptoms and smoking (people were included as smokers if they smoked in the past 2 weeks).[8] In addition, the investigators compared smokers (at least one cigarette per day) vs nonsmokers in terms of RLS symptoms and PLM in a sleep laboratory. No significant differences between the two groups were found for all sleep and motor variables. A major limitation in this study was that the smoking assessment did not account for nicotine dose, duration of habit, or degree of dependence. In contrast, association between RLS and smoking (more than one pack per day) was found in a 2000 epidemiologic study noted[6] and a 2004 study that found ex-smokers and current smokers were at higher risk for RLS.[9]

■ Considerations for Medications

Psychiatric Medications

Typical neuroleptic medications and newer atypical neuroleptic medications that are often used to treat psychiatric conditions, such as schizophrenia, bipolar disorders, and treatment-resistant depression, may worsen RLS, as they have been found to decrease dopamine neurotransmission.[10] In fact, their common side effects include akathisia, a condition that shares many clinical features with RLS.[11] While there are case reports in the medical literature that describe the onset of RLS with the typical and atypical neuroleptic medications, there have been no formal studies on these drugs to validate their effect on RLS, and many RLS patients have reported worsening symptoms while taking them.

Similar to the situation with neuroleptic drugs, there are no controlled studies validating the link between antidepressant drugs used to treat depression and anxiety and worsening RLS symptoms. There are case reports of worsening RLS while on many of the SSRIs and tricyclic antidepressants (TCAs). However, some people have improvement of their RLS symptoms while on antidepressants. This is difficult to explain in light of the many reports of exacerbation of RLS by these drugs. By improving depression and anxiety, these drugs may improve the patient's reaction to their uncomfortable symptoms much like their effect upon the discomfort from neuropathies and musculoskeletal disorders.

When neuroleptic or antidepressant medications are used to treat psychiatric disorders, it may be difficult to avoid prescribing them. Stopping or reducing them, even when RLS symptoms are clearly exacerbated, should be done with great trepidation due to concerns about worsening the underlying psychiatric disorder. *Chapter 12* discusses in detail how to manage RLS patient on neuroleptic medications.

Antihistamines

Because of their OTC availability and widespread use, antihistamines are among the most common to worsen RLS from the patient's perspective. Despite this, there are few reports describing this problem. One study found that diphenhydramine 25 mg, given intravenously, severely exacerbated RLS symptoms.[12]

Typically, it is the older, sedating antihistamines that cross the blood-brain barrier that tend to worsen RLS. Many of these are now sold OTC for control of allergy and cold symptoms.

Owing to their ubiquitous presence in combination cold and cough remedies, many people with RLS take antihistamines inadvertently and exacerbate their RLS symptoms. In addition, people suffering from RLS have trouble falling asleep and will take OTC sleeping pills that often contain one of two antihistamines: diphenhydramine or doxylamine. Afterward, RLS patients often experience increased RLS symptoms, which may then further prolong their insomnia.

Antinausea, Antiemetic, and "Antidizzy" Medications

Although there are no studies on direct association between these medications and exacerbation of RLS, there are many patients who complain of this association. Typically, RLS exacerbation occurs with the medications that ends with "-zine": promethazine, hydroxyzine, prochlorperazine, and meclizine. Also included are trimethobenzamide and dimenhydrinate. Most of them are antihistamines or neuroleptic medications used to treat nausea, emesis, and dizziness, and they typically worsen RLS. Additionally, they are all sedating drugs, which may further explain their effect on RLS.

Another antinausea drug, metoclopramide, which is a dopamine receptor antagonist, has been known to exacerbate RLS. Interestingly, in spite of frequent clinical observations, the only scientific study that examined this interaction found only a nonsignificant worsening of RLS with metoclopramide.[13]

Sedative Hypnotics

There are many other anecdotal complaints about various other medications affecting RLS aside from the ones discussed above. However, few have been noted to exacerbate RLS at any significant frequency. There are some concerns with the benzodiazepine class of sedative hypnotics that are often used to treat RLS. As a rule of thumb, any medication that induces sedation has a potential to worsen RLS. This was demonstrated in one study that reported worsening of RLS symptoms with the intravenous administration of lorazepam.[12] Although these sedatives/anxiolytic drugs may be helpful to promote sleep in RLS sufferers, they should be used with caution, especially during the daytime. Furthermore, the long-acting benzodiazepines (eg, clonazepam) may cause daytime drowsiness, which could be counterproductive for treating RLS.

There is one case report of the drug sodium oxybate, which is used for narcolepsy and cataplexy, which was given to a patient with narcolepsy, resulting in a severe new occurrence of typical RLS symptoms that resolved when the drug was discontinued.[14]

■ **RLS-Friendly Alternative Drugs**
For many of the drugs above that tend to worsen RLS, physicians can prescribe other drugs that do not affect RLS. The more friendly drugs for a number of conditions are listed in **Table 8.2**.

Sleep Hygiene

In review articles, one of the more frequently cited nonpharmacologic treatments for RLS is proper sleep hygiene.[1,15,16] Despite that, there is really no validation of this issue in the medical literature. However, it is thought that getting sufficient sleep to decrease daytime drowsiness should also diminish daytime RLS symptoms.

■ **Avoiding Sleep Deprivation**
Avoiding sleep deprivation can be a significant problem for those with RLS. As discussed in *Chapter 2*, about 70% of people with moderate to severe RLS take 30 to 60 minutes or longer to fall asleep, and 60% of them experience more than three awakenings

TABLE 8.2 — Alternatives for Dopamine-Blocking Medications for Allergy, Nausea, and Dizziness

Drugs	Comments
Alternatives for Antihistamines	
Loratadine, desloratadine, fexofenadine	These nonsedating drugs do not cross the blood-brain barrier or affect RLS
Steroid, cromolyn, and ipratropium nasal sprays, or montelukast	These are alternatives for treating rhinitis
Alternatives for Antinausea, Antiemetics, Antidizzy Drugs	
Granisetron hydrochloride, ondansetron hydrochloride, dolasetron mesylate	These newer selective 5-hydroxytryptamine receptor antagonists are used to treat the side effects of chemotherapy and do not affect RLS
Transdermal scopolamine patches	This patch is a good alternative to prevent motion sickness and does not worsen RLS
Domperidone	This drug is only available outside the United States. It acts peripherally (does not cross the blood-brain barrier) and does not affect RLS

per night. Since RLS symptoms occur most often at bedtime, it is easy to see how these symptoms interfere with obtaining sufficient sleep.

As many people need to rise at a fixed hour in order to get to work on time, the delay in sleep onset and interrupted sleep cannot be compensated by sleeping later in the morning.

Practicing proper sleep hygiene may be helpful to avoid daytime drowsiness and maintain sufficient alertness to avert an increase in RLS symptoms. The important rules of sleep hygiene that apply to those who suffer from RLS are discussed below.

■ Regular Bedtimes and Rise Times

Standardizing bedtime and wake time can be helpful in strengthening the circadian sleep-wake cycle. This task can be difficult for many RLS sufferers, since their symptoms tend to peak around bedtime. It is common for them to schedule less sedentary activities, such as cleaning the house, in the evening which will permit them to avoid being bothered by RLS symptoms. However, these active endeavors are also more alerting and are not conducive to promoting sleep. If possible, other measures (discussed below) should be implemented that may both relieve the RLS symptoms and promote natural sleepiness.

RLS symptoms follow the body's circadian rhythm, peaking in the evening/bedtime and waning throughout the sleep period until its nadir at about 10 AM.[17,18] Therefore, many people who experience bothersome RLS symptoms at night will be forced to delay their bedtime for several hours until their symptoms begin to naturally wane. Generally, the more severe the RLS, the longer it takes for the nighttime symptoms to wane sufficiently to allow sleep. Many may not be able to fall asleep before 3 AM to 6 AM, which can make it difficult to get up a few hours later for work.

Shift work usually presents challenges for patients with insomnia, who do poorly with variable bedtimes and wake times, and it may be even harder for those with insomnia induced by RLS. It may seem that the evening or night shift would be helpful for those with RLS since they could be active when symptoms tend to be maximal. This schedule may work for a few days but as the circadian rhythm resets (as this rhythm is more dependent upon the wake time), the RLS symptoms will also shift back to bedtime. The same is true for people who do not have to get up at a fixed time to work and start going to bed later and sleeping later. Within several days, they will have simply shifted their circadian cycles and RLS problems to a different time of day.

As discussed earlier, regular rise times are important to maintain proper function of the circadian rhythm. Even if people have the option of sleeping in, it is recommended that they get out of bed at the same time each day. This aspect of sleep is much easier to accomplish by simply using an alarm clock. Due to social and other pressures, it is usually more difficult to maintain a regular bedtime, especially when also being plagued by RLS symptoms that force one out of bed.

■ **Prepare the Bedroom**

Having a bedroom environment that is conducive to falling asleep is important for people with insomnia and even more so for those with RLS. Thus people with RLS should follow some of the general measures recommended for those with insomnia.

This includes controlling the temperature as well as the noise and light levels. Temperature is an individual preference and can be set accordingly. Loud snoring from bed partners, sounds of people talking, or television and traffic noises can disrupt sleep. Although these disturbances cannot always be avoided, people can employ measures to reduce their effects. White-noise generators (eg, the SoundScreen or CD players with sounds of rain, waves, wind, etc) can obscure most moderate level noises. Depending upon the time of year and location, the intrusion of daylight may interrupt sleep. Blinds, blackout curtains, or other means are recommended to keep the room dark.

142

The bed itself can be important. Movements by bed partners can easily disturb sleep. Most people with insomnia toss and turn frequently, and this is an even bigger problem for those with RLS. Due to the urge to move their legs, they usually need more room and are anxious about disturbing their bed partner. A solution to this problem is to either get twin beds (that can be separated by ½ inch at sleep time) or a king-size bed made of viscoelastic foam (such as a TempurPedic) that diminishes any movement. Bed covers and blankets can be an issue for many with RLS. Some prefer tight or heavy covers, while others cannot have any contact with their blanket.

With all of these issues that may not always have an easy alternative (ie, a bed partner snoring very loudly), it is often beneficial to have an alternate bedroom in which to sleep. Additionally, RLS sufferers may feel that they need to be completely free to move and calm their restless legs without worrying about the effect on their bed partner. It is not unusual for them to have strange sleep positions that soothe their legs enough to enable them to sleep. This includes having their feet propped up on the back of a couch or sleeping on the floor with their legs propped up against the wall.

■ Pre-sleep Activity

One of the recommendations for sleep hygiene is to establish a pre-bedtime routine that helps one unwind. This is much easier for most people with insomnia, but those with RLS usually cannot perform the sedentary activities that are relaxing while their symptoms are peaking before bedtime. In fact, relaxing may be counterproductive.

Many people with RLS choose counterstimulation techniques (see below) or other activities that calm their RLS symptoms. One of the more common counterstimulation techniques includes taking hot baths or showers. Some prefer cold water while others may alternate hot and cold water (using the bathtub faucet), running the water over their legs for 5 to 15 minutes.

Alternatively, hot or cold packs are sometimes used. This may provide a few minutes of relief, often enough to help the sleep-deprived person fall asleep.

Other common counterstimulation practices involve rubbing the legs, massages, stretches, deep knee bends, and other activities that work the leg muscles. The duration needed to get relief can vary considerably as does the interval of the relief.

Exercise

Moderate-intensity exercise has been recommended for people with insomnia as it has been shown to increase slow wave (stage 3 deep) sleep,[19] sleep duration,[20] and sleep efficiencies,[21,22] and to decrease awakenings[23] and decrease the latency to sleep onset.[24] Additionally, the timing of exercise may be important in that some studies have demonstrated that these benefits accrue only with morning exercise but not with evening exercise.[24,25] These suggestions can also be applied to those with RLS, except as noted, when their preference for evening exercise may be counterproductive.

Exercise may have other direct benefits for RLS sufferers. One study found that people with RLS showed improvement with a 12-week conditioning program of aerobic and lower-body resistance training 3 days per week compared with those who did not exercise.[23] However, this benefit seems to occur only with moderate exercise; it is common for vigorous exercise (running, training for competition, etc) to markedly worsen RLS symptoms. This may occur even when exercising strenuously in the morning, and the negative effects may last for several days.

Therefore, the best advice for patients with RLS is to exercise regularly at moderate intensity early in the day. Pre-bedtime exercise or stretching routines should be as short as possible to avoid increasing alertness and thus promoting insomnia.

Mental Alerting Activities

RLS symptoms tend to be triggered by physical or mental inactivity. Therefore, activities that promote alertness (which in turn activates the body's motor systems) may be particularly helpful to abate RLS symptoms, especially when physical movement is otherwise restricted. Situations such as travel (especially by airplane when the fasten-seat-belt sign is on), meetings, or religious services are typical examples that benefit from alerting measures.

Almost any activity that requires thinking will relieve RLS symptoms. Below is a list of common activities that help RLS:

- Playing cards, such as solitaire if alone
- Playing computer or video games
- Knitting, needlework, or other handwork
- Working on a crossword or other puzzles
- Engaging in an interesting discussion or argument
- Balancing a checkbook, homework, paperwork, or working with spreadsheets
- Writing a diary, letter, or internet blog
- Listening to music actively
- Reading an engrossing book.

As long as the person engages in these activities, the RLS symptoms will be controlled. Often, keeping mentally alert can relieve symptoms for hours, which is long enough for most domestic airplane trips. However, watching an in-flight movie is not very mentally active as it typically provides no relief.

Counterstimulation Techniques

These techniques have already been discussed somewhat in other sections, as they are useful for coping with many situations that cause RLS symptoms, especially when medication is not effective or available.

It is thought that these counterstimulation procedures work much the same way that shaking one's hand helps abate the pain from hitting a finger with a hammer.

Most of these activities are focused on the legs but also apply to other affected body parts, such as the arms:

- Hot or cold baths or showers
- Run hot or cold water on the legs (or alternate the temperatures every few minutes)
- Cold or hot packs applied to the legs
- Electric blankets
- Leg massage (manual or electrical)
- Vibration pads
- Leg tickling
- Leg wraps (eg, Ace bandages), surgical support stockings.

The duration that these techniques need to be done can be quite variable. Often a few minutes can provide long enough relief so that the RLS sufferer can go to bed and fall asleep before symptoms return and cause insomnia.

Alternative Treatments

Despite the general lack of medical evidence, many people who are frustrated with the traditional/pharmacologic treatments for RLS or other chronic conditions turn to alternative therapies. There is a broad range of remedies from which to choose. Despite their lack of proven efficacy or recommendations from traditional doctors, a large percentage of patients will seek them out. Physicians should be aware of these treatments, as patients wish to discuss them or are already using them.

■ Complementary and Alternative Medicine (CAM)

These therapies are divided into five main categories. Due to the overwhelming interest and use of CAM, the National Institutes of Health has established the National Center for Complementary and Alternative Medicine (NCCAM). Its website (*www.nccam.nih.gov*) is informative and an excellent resource for research, education, training, and news on CAM. Few scientific medical studies have examined the potential benefit of these treatments for RLS.

Alternative Medical Systems

These are separate medical systems that are built upon complete systems of theory and practice, which differ from conventional medicine. Examples include homeopathic medicine, naturopathic medicine, traditional Chinese medicine, and ayurveda (East Indian therapy based on diet and herbal remedies that emphasizes the use of body, mind, and spirit in disease prevention and treatment).

Acupuncture and acupressure are among the more common of these modalities that people seek for disorders that cause pain or discomfort. Only two articles for RLS treatment have been published so far, both in the Chinese traditional medicine literature.[26] Whether this therapy is effective outside of China remains to be determined but so far, sporadic anecdotal reports from RLS sufferers have not been very positive.

Mind-Body Interventions

This category involves techniques designed to enhance the mind's capacity to affect bodily functions and symptoms. Examples include meditation, prayer, mental healing, and therapies that use creative outlets such as art, music, or dance.

Biologically Based Therapies

These therapies use substances found in nature, such as herbs, foods, and vitamins. These are among the most popular treatments used by RLS patients and are readily purchased from health food stores, pharmacies, and on the internet.

Manipulative and Body-Based Methods

These methods are based on manipulation and/or movement of one or more parts of the body. Some examples include chiropractic or osteopathic manipulation and massage.

Energy Therapies

Biofield therapies (energy fields that purportedly surround and penetrate the human body but have never been scientifically proved) and bioelectromagnetic-based therapies (unconventional use of electromagnetic fields, such as pulsed fields, magnetic fields, or alternating-current or direct-current fields) make up this category.

■ Chiropractic Medicine

People see chiropractors for many different ailments including pain. Currently, there is only one case report[27] describing benefit from this therapy. Sporadic anecdotal reports so far do not indicate that this treatment is helpful for RLS symptoms.

■ Acupuncture and Acupressure

There have been several studies in the literature but a 2008 Cochrane Database Review[28] found that there was insufficient evidence to determine whether acupuncture is an efficacious and safe treatment for RLS. In 2011, Cripps performed a retrospective study[29] by questioning 19 RLS patients (three of whom had been on dopamine agonists) who had received acupuncture and found that they had significant improvement of their RLS symptoms based on a visual analog scale. However, in clinical practice, most patients report little or no sustained benefit from this therapy.

Surgery

In a 1995 study, Kanter[30] performed sclerotherapy with sodium tetradecyl sulphate on 113 patients with and without Doppler-proven varicose veins and found that a majority of patients improved after two treatments. At 2 years of follow-up, 28% (12 of 43) of patients who were available for follow-up had recurrence of their RLS symptoms. Hayes, in 2008, performed endovenous laser ablation and ultrasound-guided sclerotherapy in 35 patients with moderate to very severe RLS and duplex-proven superficial venous insufficiency.[31] The mean IRLS score decreased by 21.4 points (from 26.9 to 5.5) after the procedure but no long-term follow-up of these patients' symptoms is available. However, these are case-series studies only, and better designed studies (eg, sham-controlled studies) are necessary before this therapy can be recommended for RLS treatment.

There are several reports that describe worsening of RLS after surgeries. These include worsening of RLS after gastric surgery,[32] after above-knee leg amputation,[33] after heart surgery,[34] and after lung surgery.[35] The cause of surgery exacerbating RLS is unknown and may be due to multiple factors. However, it is interesting to note that there are many anecdotal reports of worsening or triggering of RLS after trauma or injury (especially spine or back related).[36] These have not been validated by formal epidemiologic studies.

There several reports of improvement for secondary RLS symptoms associated with end-stage renal disease after kidney transplantation.[37,38] RLS symptoms disappeared within 1 to 21 days of the transplant, with four of 11 patients remaining symptom-free up to 9 years, three patients had gradual reemergence of mild symptoms, and three patients in whom their transplants failed developed recurrence of RLS symptoms at their previous severity within 10 days to 2 months.

Various other surgeries have limited evidence for ameliorating RLS. These include one case report of RLS symptoms being immediately relieved postoperatively in the contralateral limbs after undergoing pallidotomy for PD.[39] Another study reported on six advanced PD patients who underwent bilateral subthalamic nucleus deep brain stimulation surgery and showed marked improvement in their RLS symptoms postoperatively.[40] However, in a study that implanted deep-brain stimulators into the ventralis intermedius nucleus of the thalamus in nine subjects for essential tremor noted that although the tremor was improved, there was no change in the concomitant RLS symptoms.[41]

Patient Organizations and Support Groups

Many patients with RLS feel isolated as if they are the only ones with the disorder. This belief is changing due to the increased awareness that RLS has received over the past few years, but it is still all too common for RLS patients to feel alone and misunderstood. Joining a patient organization or support group is one of the best ways to combat the problem of isolation, and at the same time, become more educated about the disorder through peers.

The RLS Foundation (*www.rls.org*) is an international nonprofit RLS organization based in Rochester, Minnesota, that has advocated for and helped RLS patients since its inception in 1992. Their website contains information for patients on every aspect of RLS, including a list of doctors who treat RLS. Brochures can be obtained on many RLS topics and they publish a quarterly newsletter, *NightWalkers*. They also supply a medical alert card that details the drugs that patients should avoid.

A more complete discussion of the RLS foundation resources and activities and a list of other patient support resources can be found in Appendix B.

REFERENCES

1. Stiasny K, Oertel W H, Trenkwalder C. Clinical symptomatology and treatment of restless legs syndrome and periodic limb movement disorder. *Sleep Med Rev.* 2002;6:253-265.

2. Lutz EG. Restless legs, anxiety and caffeinism. *J Clin Psychiatry.* 1978;39:693-698.

3. Leutgeb U, Martus P. Regular intake of non-opioid analgesics is associated with an increased risk of restless legs syndrome in patients maintained on antidepressants. *Eur J Med Res.* 2002; 7:368-378.

4. Rouhani S, Tran G, Leplaideur F, Durlach J, Poenaru S. EEG effects of a single low dose of ethanol on afternoon sleep in the nonalcohol-dependent adult. *Alcohol.* 1989;6:687-690.

5. Roth T, Roehrs T, Zorick F, Conway W. Pharmacological effects of sedative-hypnotics, narcotic analgesics, and alcohol during sleep. *Med Clin North Am.* 1985;69:1281-1288.

6. Phillips B, Young T, Finn L, Asher K, Hening WA, Purvis C. Epidemiology of restless legs symptoms in adults. *Arch Intern Med.* 2000;160:2137-2141.

7. Mountifield JA. Restless leg syndrome relieved by cessation of smoking. *CMAJ.* 1985;133:426-427.

8. Lavigne GL, Lobbezoo F, Rompre PH, Nielsen TA, Montplaisir J. Cigarette smoking as a risk factor or an exacerbating factor for restless legs syndrome and sleep bruxism. *Sleep.* 1997;20:290-293.

9. Berger K, Luedemann J, Trenkwalder C, John U, Kessler C. Sex and the risk of restless legs syndrome in the general population. *Arch Intern Med.* 2004;164:196-202.

10. Chiodo LA. Dopamine-containing neurons in the mammalian central nervous system: electrophysiology and pharmacology. *Neurosci Biobehav Rev.* 1988;12:49-91.

11. Walters AS, Hening W, Rubinstein M, Chokroverty S. A clinical and polysomnographic comparison of neuroleptic-induced akathisia and the idiopathic restless legs syndrome. *Sleep.* 1991;14:339-345.

12. Allen RP, Lesage S, Earley CJ. Anti-histamines and benzodiazepines exacerbate daytime restless legs syndrome (RLS) symptoms. *Sleep.* 2005;28:A279. Abstract.

13. Winkelmann J, Schadrack J, Wetter TC, Zieglgansberger W, Trenkwalder C. Opioid and dopamine antagonist drug challenges in untreated restless legs syndrome patients. *Sleep Med.* 2001;2:57-61.

8

14. Abril B, Carlander B, Touchon J, Dauvilliers Y. Restless legs syndrome in narcolepsy: a side effect of sodium oxybate? *Sleep Med.* 2007;8:181-183.

15. Paulson GW. Restless legs syndrome. How to provide symptom relief with drug and nondrug therapies. *Geriatrics.* 2000;55:35-38.

16. Hening W, Allen R, Earley C, Kushida C, Picchietti D, Silber M. The treatment of restless legs syndrome and periodic limb movement disorder. An American Academy of Sleep Medicine Review. *Sleep.* 1999;22:970-999.

17. Trenkwalder C, Hening WA, Walters AS, Campbell SS, Rahman K, Chokroverty S. Circadian rhythm of periodic limb movements and sensory symptoms of restless legs syndrome. *Mov Disord.* 1999;14:102-110.

18. Hening WA, Walters AS, Wagner M, et al. Circadian rhythm of motor restlessness and sensory symptoms in the idiopathic restless legs syndrome. *Sleep.* 1999;22:901-912.

19. Naylor E, Penev PD, Orbeta L, et al. Daily social and physical activity increases slow-wave sleep and daytime neuropsychological performance in the elderly. *Sleep.* 2000;23:87-95.

20. King AC, Oman RF, Brassington GS, Bliwise DL, Haskell WL. Moderate-intensity exercise and self-rated quality of sleep in older adults. A randomized controlled trial. *JAMA.* 1997; 277:32-37.

21. Norman JF, Von Essen SG, Fuchs RH, McElligott M. Exercise training effect on obstructive sleep apnea syndrome. *Sleep Res Online.* 2000;3:121-129.

22. Shapiro CM, Warren PM, Trinder J, et al. Fitness facilitates sleep. *Eur J Appl Physiol Occup Physiol.* 1984;53:1-4.

23. Aukerman MM, Aukerman D, Bayard M, Tudiver F, Thorp L, Bailey B. Exercise and restless legs syndrome: a randomized controlled trial. *J Am Board Fam Med.* 2006;19:487-493.

24. Youngstedt SD, O'Connor PJ, Dishman RK. The effects of acute exercise on sleep: a quantitative synthesis. *Sleep.* 1997; 20:203-214.

25. Tworoger SS, Yasui Y, Vitiello MV, et al. Effects of a yearlong moderate-intensity exercise and a stretching intervention on sleep quality in postmenopausal women. *Sleep.* 2003;26:830-836.

26. Hu J. Acupuncture treatment of restless leg syndrome. *J Tradit Chin Med.* 2001;21:312-316.

27. Stupar MJ. Restless legs syndrome in a primary contact setting: a case report. *Can Chiropr Assoc.* 2008;52(2):81-87.

28. Cui Y, Wang Y, Liu Z. Acupuncture for restless legs syndrome. *Cochrane Database Syst Rev.* 2008;(4):CD006457.

29. Cripps MG. Acupuncture for restless legs syndrome in patients previously treated with dopaminergic drugs. *Acupunct Med.* 2011;29(3):240-241.

30. Kanter AH. The effect of sclerotherapy on restless legs syndrome. *Dermatol Surg.* 1995;21(4):328-332.

31. Hayes CA, Kingsley JR, Hamby KR, Carlow J. The effect of endovenous laser ablation on restless legs syndrome. *Phlebology.* 2008;23(3):112-117.

32. Banerji NK, Hurwitz LJ. Restless legs syndrome, with particular reference to its occurrence after gastric surgery. *Br Med J.* 1970;4:774-775.

33. Hanna PA, Kumar S, Walters AS. Restless legs symptoms in a patient with above knee amputations: a case of phantom restless legs. *Clin Neuropharmacol.* 2004;27:87-89.

34. Cortese S, Konofal E, Lecendreux M, Mouren MC, Bernardina BD. Restless legs syndrome triggered by heart surgery. *Pediatr Neurol.* 2006;35:223-226.

35. Minai OA, Golish JA, Yataco JC, Budev MM, Blazey H, Giannini C. Restless legs syndrome in lung transplant recipients. *J Heart Lung Transplant.* 2007;26:24-29.

36. Walters AS, Wagner M, Hening WA. Periodic limb movements as the initial manifestation of restless legs syndrome triggered by lumbosacral radiculopathy. *Sleep.* 1996;19:825-826.

37. Yasuda T, Nishimura A, Katsuki Y, Tsuji Y. Restless legs syndrome treated successfully by kidney transplantation—a case report. *Clin Transpl.* 1986:138.

38. Winkelmann J, Stautner A, Samtleben W, Trenkwalder C. Long-term course of restless legs syndrome in dialysis patients after kidney transplantation. *Mov Disord.* 2002;17:1072-1076.

39. Rye DB, DeLong MR. Amelioration of sensory limb discomfort of restless legs syndrome by pallidotomy. *Ann Neurol.* 1999; 46:800-801.

40. Driver-Dunckley E, Evidente VG, Adler CH, et al. Restless legs syndrome in Parkinson's disease patients may improve with subthalamic stimulation. *Mov Disord.* 2006;21:1287-1289.

41. Ondo W. VIM deep brain stimulation does not improve pre-existing restless legs syndrome in patients with essential tremor. *Parkinsonism Relat Disord.* 2006;12:113-114.

8

9
Pharmacologic Management

When nonpharmacologic therapy is no longer adequate, treatment with drugs should be strongly considered (as discussed in *Chapter 7*). There are now four FDA-approved RLS drugs in the United States, which makes the choice of treatment more complicated. In addition, there are many drugs not approved by the FDA that are effective for treating RLS and should be available in the arsenal of doctors who are treating RLS. The recently published American Academy of Sleep Medicine (AASM) Clinical Practice Guideline on the treatment of RLS and PLM provides an excellent overview of the current evidence for pharmacotherapy of moderate-to-severe RLS based on rigorous systematic review and meta-analyses.[1] However, this guideline does not include a recommendation for rotigotine, a transdermal patch newly FDA-approved for the treatment of moderate-to-severe RLS. This chapter will comprehensively review all the medications that have been studied for relieving RLS and discuss their use, including benefits and disadvantages.

In general, there are four classes of drugs that are most useful in treating RLS (**Table 9.1**):
- Dopaminergics
- Anticonvulsants
- Opioids
- Sedative hypnotics.

Dopaminergic Medications

The first dopaminergic medication used in RLS treatment was L-dopa. L-dopa is a precursor drug in that it is enzymatically modified by dopa decarboxylase into the active neurotransmitter, dopamine. An L-dopa–containing drug was the first dopaminergic used to treat RLS in modern times by Sevket Akpinar,

TABLE 9.1 — Drug Classes Used in RLS

Dopaminergics
- Levodopa combined with a decarboxylase inhibitor
- Dopamine agonists:
  – Ropinirole
  – Pramipexole
  – Rotigotine patch

Anticonvulsants
- α2δ ligands:
  – Gabapentin enacarbil
  – Pregabalin
  – Gabapentin
- Others (non-α2δ ligands)

Opioids
- Mild, moderate, and strong for different situations

Sedative hypnotics
- Benzodiazepines
- Nonbenzodiazepines

a Turkish neurologist, in 1982.[2] When RLS patients started taking L-dopa, it was as if their troublesome symptoms were magically relieved. However, after an initial dramatic period of relief, the majority who took these drugs on a daily basis began experiencing a marked worsening of their RLS symptoms (called augmentation, *see below*).[3] Due to this problem of augmentation, it is recommended that L-dopa should not be used on a daily basis. This finding has led to the registration of dopamine agonists for RLS with ropinirole (May 2005), pramipexole (November 2006), and the rotigotine transdermal patch (April 2012) being approved by the FDA in the United States. All dopaminergic drugs have been at least temporarily effective in RLS and all share a spectrum of adverse effects. These are detailed in **Table 9.2**. Individual drugs may be more or less associated with specific side effects, as discussed below.

TABLE 9.2 — Dopaminergic Side Effects

Common Acute Adverse Effects
- Nausea; less commonly, vomiting
- Light headedness; rarely, syncope
- Headache
- Somnolence
- Insomnia

Less Common Adverse Effects
- Peripheral edema
- Sleep attacks
- Impulse control disorders:
  - Hypersexuality
  - Pathologic gambling
  - Excessive shopping
  - Punding

Subacute to Late Onset Adverse Effects
- Augmentation:
  - Advance in time of onset of symptoms
  - Greater severity of symptoms when present
  - Reduced latency to onset of symptoms at rest
  - Spread of symptoms to involve new body parts

Adverse Effects Primarily Shown in Parkinson's Disease
- Dyskinesias
- Hallucinations
- Psychosis

Adverse Effects Associated With Ergoline Derivatives
- Fibrotic syndromes
  - Retroperitoneal fibrosis
  - Pleuropulmonary fibrosis
  - Fibrotic cardiomyopathy

Adverse Effects Associated With Transdermal Dopaminergics
- Application site reaction

Dopamine Agonists

Dopamine agonists have until recently been considered as the sole drugs of choice for daily RLS symptoms.[4] Before gabapentin enacarbil was approved by the FDA (April 2011), they were the only drugs that were approved for treatment of idiopathic RLS in both Europe and the United States. Physicians should become familiar with these drugs and be comfortable using them to treat RLS. Currently, two short-acting (pramipexole and ropinirole) and one long-acting (rotigotine transdermal patch) dopamine agonists are approved for treating RLS. **Table 9.3** lists the dopamine agonists and their usual doses.

■ Approved Medications *(in alphabetical order)*

Pramipexole

Pramipexole was the second drug approved by the FDA for the treatment of moderate-to-severe primary RLS in the United States. Similar to ropinirole, many studies have confirmed its efficacy in RLS.[5-10] Two large ($n = 344$ or 345) double-blinded, placebo-controlled trials evaluated efficacy and safety of pramipexole treatment of primary RLS, with a randomization giving twice as many subjects on pramipexole as placebo. The primary end points in both studies were the clinical global improvement and the change from baseline in IRLS scores. The European study,[10] with individually titrated doses ranging from 0.125 or 0.75 (median pramipexole dose of 0.35 mg/day), reported a positive response after 6 weeks of treatment. The mean IRLS score decreases were 5.7 for placebo and 12.3 for pramipexole. The percentage of "much/very much improved" ratings was 32.5% on placebo and 62.9% on pramipexole (**Figure 9**.1).

In the second study conducted in the United States,[8] patients were randomized to receive a placebo or one of three fixed pramipexole doses: 0.25, 0.5, or 0.75 mg/day. Responses at 12 weeks showed decreases on the IRLS of 9.3 for placebo vs 12.8 for 0.25 mg pramipexole, 13.8 for 0.5 mg, and 14.1 for 0.75 mg (**Figure 9**.1). The percentage of "much/very much improved" on the CGI scale was 51.2% for placebo vs 74.7% for 0.25 pramipexole, 67.9% for 0.5 mg, and 72.9% for 0.75 mg. In addition, 150 RLS patients who had responded to pramipexole were then randomly switched to either placebo or continuing on

TABLE 9.3 — Dopamine Agonists

Generic Drug Name	Half-Life in Hours	Route Metabolized or Eliminated	Ergot Alkaloid Derivative	Doses per Day	Individual Dose Range (mg)	Average Daily Dose (mg)	Approved for Treating RLS
Apomorphine (subcutaneous)	½-1	Unknown	No	1-?	?	?	No
Bromocriptine	3-12	Liver	Yes	1-3	2.5-10	10-15	No
Cabergoline	>65	Liver	Yes	1	0.25-4	1.5-2	No
Lisuride	2-3	Liver	Yes	1	0.1-0.4	0.3	No
Pergolide	7-16	Liver	Yes	1-3	0.05-1.0	0.25-0.5	No
Piribedil (sustained release)	21	?	No	1	25-350	50-150	No
Pramipexole	8-12	Kidney	No	1-3	0.125-1.5	0.125-0.25	Yes
Ropinirole	6	Liver	No	1-3	0.25-4	0.25-1	Yes
Rotigotine (transdermal)	3 initial, 5-7 terminal	Liver, then excreted by the kidneys	No	1	1-3	1-3	Yes
Terguride	4	Kidney	Yes	1-3	0.25-0.75	0.5	No

9

FIGURE 9.1 — Efficacy of Pramipexole: IRLS

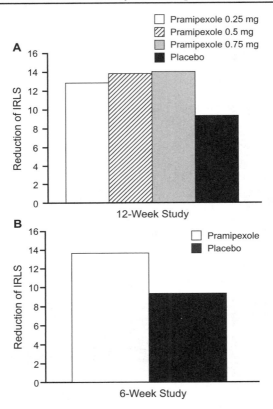

A) This was a 12-week fixed-dose trial of pramipexole in comparison with placebo.[1] There was a significant reduction of the IRLS summed score at each dose level. *B)* This was a 6-week flexible-dose study of pramipexole compared with placebo.[2] There was a significant reduction of the IRLS summed score; mean pramipexole dose at measurement was 0.35 mg/day.

[1] Winkelman JW, et al. *Neurology*. 2006;67:1034-1039.
[2] Oertel WH, et al. *Mov Disord*. 2007;22:213-219.

their pramipexole and followed this treatment course for another 3 months.[7] The percentage of patients with predefined worsening of their RLS symptoms and also a decrease in CGI was 85.5% for placebo and 20.5% for pramipexole treatment.

A third study was a dose-finding parallel-group PSG study in which a total of 109 patients were randomly administered one of the following: placebo, 0.125 mg, 0.25 mg, 0.5 mg, or 0.75 mg for 3 weeks.[6] The PLMI was reduced in all four drug groups by about 80% compared with placebo (**Figure 9.2**). The IRLS score was lower for all drug doses compared with placebo, with the higher doses showing >50% reduction.[6] In summary, these three large clinical trials showed that pramipexole is efficacious in RLS at doses ranging from 0.25 to 0.75 mg per day (**Figure 9.1**). These studies also provided evidence that pramipexole improved sleep and quality of life in RLS patients.

As noted in **Table 9.3**, pramipexole has a half-life of 8 to 12 hours (for young to older subjects) and is excreted through the kidneys. Drugs that are inhibitors of renal tubular secretion of organic bases via the cationic transport system (eg, cimetidine, ranitidine, diltiazem, triamterene, verapamil, quinidine, and quinine) decrease the elimination of pramipexole.

Pramipexole is approved for use in moderate to severe primary RLS once daily at 2 to 3 hours before bedtime. It has been used off-label up to three times daily (2 to 3 hours before the onset of symptoms) for patients with symptoms that occur substantially before bedtime. Its onset of effective action is a little slower than that of ropinirole, taking 2 to 3 hours to reach optimal effect. Like ropinirole, it is fully absorbed with food but will then have a 1-hour delay in its onset of action.

Typically, pramipexole should be started at 0.125 mg, then can be increased by 0.125 mg every 5 to 7 days to a maximum of 0.5 mg until RLS symptoms are relieved. More gradual titration schedules tend to limit side effects. Although the FDA has approved a

9

FIGURE 9.2 — Efficacy of Pramipexole: PLM

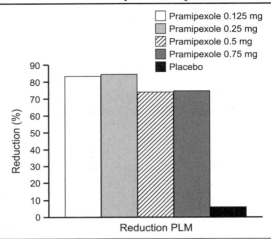

This study was a 3-week fixed-dose study using pramipexole doses from 0.125 to 0.75 mg compared with placebo. Reduction of periodic limb movement index, both awake and asleep, was significant at each dose level.

Partinen M, et al. *Sleep Med.* 2006;7:407-417.

maximum dose of 0.5 mg, many RLS experts think that lower doses may be safer in the long run (see the discussion of augmentation below). Therefore, it may be prudent to not exceed 0.25 mg but rather add another class of drug if symptoms are not relieved. Elderly patients (over 70 to 75 years old) may respond to lower doses and can be started at one half of a 0.125 mg tablet, and even incremented by that dose every 5 to 7 days as needed.

Although only FDA approved for once-daily use, pramipexole is sometimes used off-label two or even three times daily (administered 1 to 2 hours before the onset of symptoms) to treat RLS symptoms that occur earlier in the day. However, using this drug more than once daily should be done with caution as the resultant higher dose levels increase the chances of side effects (especially augmentation).

Adverse reactions are similar to the dopamine side effects listed in **Table 9**.**2**.

Ropinirole

Ropinirole was the first dopamine agonist approved in the United States (May 2005) by the FDA for treating moderate-to-severe primary RLS. It was later approved in Europe. Several studies have confirmed the efficacy of this drug in RLS treatment.[11-14] The three major trials followed similar methodology as the studies listed above. Each trial lasted 12 weeks, with the dose of ropinirole being titrated upward in an unforced paradigm from 0.25 mg to a maximum of 4 mg administered in a single dose 1 to 3 hours before bed. The primary end point was the IRLS in two studies[11,12] and the PLMI on PSG in the third study.[13] The mean dose used in the three studies was 1.8 or 1.9 mg. The IRLS scores were significantly lower with ropinirole compared with placebo. The degree of difference between the placebo and treatment groups was 3.0[11] and 2.5.[12] In the third study, ropinirole resulted in a significant 70% decrease in PLMS and 61% decrease in PLMW compared with the placebo.[13] In summary, ropinirole provided both a subjective benefit to patients with RLS (**Figure 9**.**3**) and reduced their involuntary movements (PLM) at night (**Figure 9**.**4**). Additional measures of sleep and quality of life also showed greater benefit with ropinirole than with placebo in these studies.

As noted in **Table 9**.**3**, this drug has a half-life of 6 hours and is metabolized in the liver. Ropinirole does not affect the metabolism of other drugs but its metabolism is slowed by inhibitors of CYP1A2, such as ciprofloxacin, and by estrogens.

Ropinirole is approved for use in moderate to severe primary RLS with once-daily dosing to treat bedtime symptoms. As the drug may take 1 to 3 hours to exert its clinical effects, it should be taken 1 to 3

9

FIGURE 9.3 — Efficacy of Ropinirole: IRLS

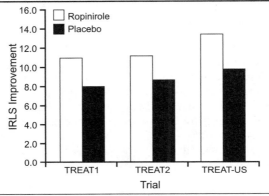

The reduction in the IRLS is given for ropinirole and placebo in three flexible dose studies: TREAT1,[1] TREAT2,[2] and TREAT-US.[3] All studies lasted 12 weeks. Mean doses at the time of measurements were: 1.9, 1.5, and 2.1 mg/day, respectively. Each trial showed a significant reduction of the IRLS score in the ropinirole group compared with placebo.

[1] Trenkwalder C, et al. *J Neurol Neurosurg Psychiatry.* 2004;75: 92-97.
[2] Walters AS, et al. *Mov Disord.* 2004;19:1414-1423.
[3] Bogan RK, et al. *Mayo Clin Proc.* 2006;81:17-27.

hours before bedtime. However, some people may benefit from its effects in as fast as 30 minutes.

Ropinirole should be started at its lowest dose of 0.25 mg and then titrated slowly (every 5 to 7 days) as necessary. Although many physicians will increase the dose by 0.5 mg or even 1 mg, it may be prudent to increase by increments of 0.25 mg. The FDA-approved maximum dose is 4 mg but as discussed above for pramipexole, not exceeding 1 mg per day may reduce the odds of side effects. Similar to pramipexole, it is sometimes used off-label two or three times per day, which also should be done with caution. Elderly patients (over 70 to 75 years old) may respond to lower doses starting with one half of a 0.25-mg tablet and incrementing by this dose every 5 to 7 days.

FIGURE 9.4 — Efficacy of Ropinirole: PLM

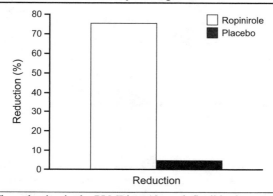

The reduction in the PLMI in a 12-week flexible-dose comparison of ropinirole to placebo. Mean dose of ropinirole at the end of the study was 1.8 mg.

Allen R, et al. *Sleep*. 2004;27:907-914.

9

Rotigotine

Rotigotine is the third dopamine agonist approved in the United States for treating moderate-to-severe RLS. It had been approved in May 2007 for PD but due to problems with precipitation of the drug resulting in crystal formation on the patch, it was removed from the US market in April 2008. The drug was reformulated and approved again in April 2012 for both RLS and PD.

Due to its very low oral bioavailability from an extensive first-pass effect, this non–ergot-derived dopamine agonist is given by the transdermal route (**Figure 9.5**). After the patch is applied, there is a lag time of about 2 to 3 hours before the drug reaches the systemic circulation and typically about 15 to 18 hours until it reaches peak concentrations (but may take up to 27 hours). Plasma levels are stable (steady state) at 2 to 3 days. After removal of the patch, plasma levels decreased with a half-life of 5 to 7 hours. Rotigotine is metabolized in the liver and then excreted mostly through the kidneys.

FIGURE 9.5 — Composition of a Rotigotine Patch

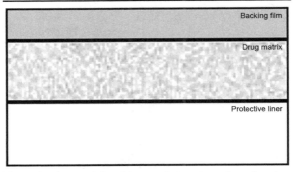

The rotigotine patch is a thin, matrix-type transdermal system composed of three layers: backing film, drug matrix, and protective liner.

The first pilot study randomized subjects with moderate to severe RLS to three patch doses: 0.5 mg, 1 mg, and 2 mg daily for 1 week.[15] All doses improved RLS symptoms, with the 2-mg dose being the most effective. The next study examined the dose-response curve with respect to safety and tolerability and optimum dosing of the rotigotine patch in a 6-week study.[16] Using five patch doses (0.5, 1, 2, 3, and 4 mg), this study found that the optimal dose range was 1 to 3 mg, as the lowest dose of 0.5 mg was not effective and there was no additional benefit with the highest dose of 4 mg.

A 6-month trial by Trenkwalder and associates in 458 patients with moderate-to-severe idiopathic RLS (average baseline IRLS sum score 28.1) randomized patients to receive placebo or transdermal rotigotine 1 mg, 2 mg, or 3 mg over 24 hours.[17] Patients began treatment at a daily dosage of 1 mg/24 hours, then were titrated over a 3-week period to their assigned dose, followed by a 6-month maintenance period. Co-primary efficacy end points were change from baseline to end of maintenance in IRLS sum score and in the clinical global impressions (CGI) item 1 score. Mean changes in IRLS sum scores from baseline to the end of the maintenance phase were significantly greater (P <0.0001) with all three dosages of rotigotine than with placebo (**Figure 9.6**). Similarly, mean changes in CGI item 1 scores from baseline to the end of the maintenance phase also were significantly greater (P

FIGURE 9.6 — Change From Baseline to the End of Maintenance for the Four Treatment Groups (Full Analysis Set, LOCF)

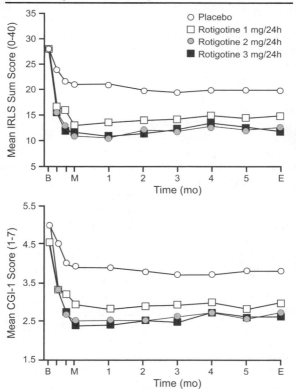

Key: B, baseline; CGI-1, Clinical Global Impressions score (item 1); E, end of maintenance phase; IRLS, International Restless Legs Scale; M, start of maintenance phase.

Trenkwalder C, et al. *Lancet Neurol*. 2008;7:595-604.

<0.0001) with all three dosages of rotigotine compared with placebo. During the titration period, onset of therapeutic effect was seen with the 1 mg/24-hour dose. Of the rotigotine-treated patients, 24% had an IRLS score of 0 at the end of the maintenance period compared with 12% of placebo patients. Ten patients had serious rotigotine-related adverse events: elevation of liver enzymes ($n=1$), worsening of tinnitus ($n=1$), nonresponse to anticoagulation ($n=1$), ECG changes ($n=1$), and application-site reactions ($n=6$). The application-site reactions all resolved within a short time of patch removal without any other intervention. The rate of typical dopaminergic side effects in patients who received rotigotine was low.

In a 6-month, placebo-controlled trial by Hening and colleagues, 505 patients with moderate to severe RLS (IRLS sum score ≥15) were assigned to five groups to receive either placebo or rotigotine (0.5, 1, 2, or 3 mg/24 hour) delivered by once-daily transdermal patch.[18] Patients began treatment at a daily dosage of 0.5 mg/24 hours, then were titrated over a 4-week period to their assigned dose, followed by a 6-month maintenance period. The co-primary efficacy end points were change from baseline to end of maintenance in IRLS sum score and in the clinical global impressions (CGI) item 1 score. At the end of the 6-month maintenance period, decreases from baseline in the two co-primary efficacy parameters were significantly greater with the 2 mg/24-hour and 3 mg/24-hour doses of rotigotine compared with placebo (**Table 9.4**). During the titration period, onset of therapeutic effect was seen with the 1 mg/24-hour dose. Of the rotigotine-treated patients, 23% had an IRLS score of 0 at the end of the maintenance period compared with 9.1% of placebo patients. Skin reactions (27%) and known dopaminergic side effects such as nausea (18.1%) and headache (11.6%) were mostly mild to moderate in rotigotine-treated patients.

Impulse control disorders (ICD), which have been documented in RLS patients taking other dopamine

TABLE 9.4 — Change From Baseline to End of Maintenance in IRLA and CGI Scores With Rotigotine or Placebo

Variable	Treatment	Mean Change From Baseline	Difference From Placebo
IRLA sum score	Placebo	−9.0	—
	Rotigotine 0.5 mg/24 hr	−11.1	
	Rotigotine 1 mg/24 hr	−11.2	
	Rotigotine 2 mg/24 hr	−13.5	
	Rotigotine 3 mg/24 hr	−14.2	
CGI Item 1	Placebo	−1.4	
	Rotigotine 0.5 mg/24 hr	−1.8	
	Rotigotine 1 mg/24 hr	−1.7	
	Rotigotine 2 mg/24 hr	−2.1	
	Rotigotine 3 mg/24 hr	−2.1	

[a] P <0.001 vs placebo.

Hening WA, et al. *Mov Disord.* 2010;25:1675-1683.

agonist drugs, have also been
with one prospective study[19]
oped signs of ICD (as m
Screening Questionnai
initiation of treatmen
and ICD behavior
ity, compulsiv
punding. (P
complex
tive a
co

oted with rotigotine,
finding that 21% devel-
easured using the Zurich
e for ICD) prior to and after
t. The mean dose was 3.8 mg/day
included binge eating, hypersexual-
e shopping, pathologic gambling, and
nding is behavior that is characterized by
, stereotyped, and often purposeless repeti-
ctions such as continued handling or sorting of
hmon objects, manipulation of technical equipment,
excessive grooming or cleaning, and hoarding. The
activity serves no purpose but is comforting and other
examples include taking apart watches or radios and
lining up pebbles.) Therefore, as with all dopamine
agonist drugs, patients on rotigotine should be frequently screened for the development of an ICD (for
further discussion of ICD, see below).

Rotigotine transdermal patches should be started
at 1 mg/24 hours and increased if needed on a weekly
basis by 1 mg/24 hours to a maximum of 3 mg/24
hours. The patch should be applied to undamaged,
non-oily skin (front of the abdomen, thigh, hip, flank,
shoulder, or upper arm) at the same time once a day
and pressed firmly in place for 30 seconds making sure
that good contact is achieved. Care should be taken
not to use the same site more than once every 14 days
to avoid irritating the skin. No dosage adjustment is
necessary for patients who have moderate impairment
of hepatic function or mild to severe impairment of
renal function.

Rotigotine is a good choice for patients with
moderate to severe RLS symptoms. It may cause
fewer problems with augmentation than the shorter-
acting dopamine agonists (pramipexole, ropinirole). It
certainly is a better option for patients who complain
of RLS symptoms that occur several hours before
bedtime and especially for symptoms that begin in the
morning. However, as discussed in *Chapter 7*, many
RLS patients with daytime symptoms simply change

170

their lifestyles to avoid sedentary situations that trigger their daytime RLS symptoms and will thus not mention them or complain about them. Despite their lack of complaints, treating their daytime symptoms with a long-acting drug such as rotigotine transdermal may provide them with a better quality of life and enable them to take advantage of work and leisure daytime sedentary activities.

Adverse effects are similar to other dopamine agonists discussed below and in **Table 9.2**, with the notable exception of skin reactions, which occurred in 39% of patients on the 3 mg/24 hour patch. The application site reactions increased with the dose and resulted in discontinuation of the drug in 12% of patients. The reactions present as localized erythema, edema, or pruritus limited to the patch area and usually do not lead to dose reduction and typically resolve within a few days after the patch is removed.

Adverse Dopamine Side Effects

Adverse effects of pramipexole, ropinirole, rotigotine transdermal, and the dopaminergic drugs are outlined in **Table 9.2**. Most of these adverse effects are common to all dopamine drugs. The most frequent side effect is nausea that tends to occur when initiating these drugs or with increasing their dose. Generally, the nausea lasts only several hours after a dose and may cease after a few days on a stable dose. Taking the medication with food (except for rotigotine which is unaffected by food intake) often mitigates the nausea but delays the onset of action by about 1 hour. Other common adverse reactions include somnolence, vomiting, dizziness, fatigue, postural hypotension, and insomnia. Some people have to discontinue the medication due to these problems but most can maintain treatment, as the reactions are often transient and mild.

The package insert warns about an increased risk of melanoma. However, this is due to the increased incidence of melanoma with PD, even though no dopamine agonist has yet been linked to melanoma. Occasional reports of hallucinations have also been noted with these drugs during RLS treatment, but these are much more common with the higher doses used for PD.

ICDS were first noted in patients with PD on dopamine agonists.[20-22] These compulsive behaviors include pathologic gambling, hypersexuality, compulsive shopping, compulsive eating, compulsive medication use, and punding. Although they were thought to occur only with the higher doses used for PD, they were subsequently documented with the lower doses employed for RLS patients.[23-25] The prevalence of this disorder is still not known but Cornelius[26] found some evidence of an ICD in 17% of RLS patients who were on a mean dose of 1.25 mg of pramipexole or 3.6 mg of ropinirole. The mean duration of onset was 9.5 months after starting therapy.

Ondo[27] found that 20% of 300 PD and RLS patients that he studied had some evidence of increased impulsivity, but only 11 out of 59 respondents thought that this behavior was deleterious. Patients tend not to report their ICD-related symptoms to their clinicians, and the underreporting makes ICD very difficult to diagnose. However, it is crucial to identify the ICD as it may result in catastrophic financial loss from gambling or destruction of personal and family relationships (eg, impulsive acts, decisions, and hypersexuality). Patients and their family should be questioned about possible ICD behaviors frequently while on dopamine agonist therapy. Symptoms will often resolve with a reduction of dose or, if necessary, complete tapering of the offending dopamine agonist.

There have been warnings about sudden sleep attacks associated with dopamine agonists. Although it is more common with the higher doses prescribed for PD, sleep attacks may still occur at the lower doses prescribed for RLS. Clinicians should apprise patients of all of these potential risks and have them start these medications on days when they do not have to drive so that this side effect can be safely assessed.

Rebound and augmentation are two problems of extended treatment. The features of these issues are given in **Table 9**.**5** and discussed below (after the L-dopa section).

TABLE 9.5 — Max Planck Institute Diagnostic Criteria for Augmentation[a]

A. Basic features (all of which need to be met):
- The increase in symptom severity experienced on 5 out of 7 days during the previous week
- The increase in symptom severity not accounted for by other factors, such as a change in medical status, lifestyle, or the natural progression of the disorder
- It is assumed that there has been a prior positive response to treatment

In addition to A, either B or C (or both) need to be satisfied.

B. Persisting (although not immediate) paradoxical response to treatment:
- RLS symptom severity increases some time after a dose increase and improves some time after a dose decrease.

C. Earlier onset of symptoms:
- An earlier onset by at least 4 hours OR
- An earlier onset (between 2 and 4 hours) occurs with one of the following compared with symptom status before treatment:
  - Shorter latency to symptoms when at rest
  - Extension of symptoms to other body parts
  - Greater intensity of symptoms or increase in periodic limb movements if measured by PSG or the SIT
  - Shorter duration of relief from treatment

[a] Augmentation requires that criteria A + B, A + C, or A+(B+C) be met.

Garcia-Borreguero D, et al. *Sleep Med*. 2007;8:520-530.

■ L-Dopa

Varied Formulations

There are currently two available forms of L-dopa: combined with carbidopa in the United States (approved only for treating PD and not for RLS) and combined with benserazide outside the United

States (approved in Europe for the treatment of RLS). Carbidopa and benserazide act only outside the central nervous system to inhibit the enzyme dopa decarboxylase from converting L-dopa into dopamine, thus decreasing the peripheral side effects and increasing the amount of L-dopa available in the brain, which reduces the required dose.

The immediate-release formulations of L-dopa may have an onset as quickly as 15 to 30 minutes on an empty stomach, which makes them useful for unexpected episodes of RLS that need rapid relief. However, these immediate-release drugs have a very short half-life of 1.5 hours and an effective duration of about 2 to 3 hours. The slow-release formulations of L-dopa (CR) may last 4 to 6 hours but have a much slower onset of action.

The side effects of L-dopa are similar to the other dopamine drugs (**Table 9.2**).

The dose range of L-dopa for RLS is 50 to 200 mg/day (combined with either 10, 25, or 50 mg carbidopa or 12.5, 25, or 50 mg benserazide). Keeping the dose <200 mg/day may help prevent augmentation, but even these smaller doses have been associated with this side effect. It is therefore best to limit the use of this drug for intermittent RLS symptoms for which it can be very useful and safe.

Extending L-dopa With COMT Inhibitors

Catechol-*O*–methyl transferase (COMT) is an enzyme that is involved in the breakdown of the catecholamine neurotransmitters, dopamine, epinephrine, and norepinephrine. This enzyme also breaks down L-dopa and, in the presence of a decarboxylase inhibitor (carbidopa or benserazide), COMT becomes the major metabolizing enzyme for L-dopa.

Therefore, adding an inhibitor of COMT to the combination medication of L-dopa and carbidopa or benserazide increases the bioavailability of L-dopa by about 2-fold. The half-life of L-dopa is increased, which results in more sustained plasma levels of the drug but the peak concentration is unaltered.

There are currently two COMT inhibitors available in the United States:

- Tolcapone
- Entacapone.

While tolcapone increases the bioavailability of L-dopa 2-fold and the half-life to 3.5 hours, entacapone increases the bioavailability of L-dopa by 35% and the half-life to 2.4 hours. However, due to the 10- to 100-fold increase in fulminant liver failure caused by tolcapone, it has been withdrawn from many countries, except the United States. There is also one combination medication that contains L-dopa, carbidopa, and tolcapone.

The use of COMT inhibitors has been well established for treating PD. However, as the use of L-dopa is now mostly limited to treating intermittent RLS symptoms, the role of adding a COMT inhibitor is an unknown. As the addition of a COMT inhibitor does not affect the time of onset or of peak concentration, these may be useful drugs to prolong the otherwise short-lived effects of L-dopa. However, until these drugs are studied, we do not really know their efficacy for treating RLS or whether they alter L-dopa's common problem of augmentation.

■ Rebound

Rebound, first described in 1993,[28] is a problem that may occur with any of the dopaminergic medications, especially the shorter-acting drugs. Rebound occurs when the effect of the drug wears off and RLS symptoms recur due to drug levels that are inadequate to control them. This is simply an end of the drug-dose effect.

A typical example of this phenomenon is the use of L-dopa (half-life of 1.5 hours) to treat bedtime RLS. If the drug is taken at 11 PM and the person wakes up after 3 AM, the low levels of drug left in the body are insufficient to relieve the reemerging RLS symptoms.

Rebound is easily managed. As soon as symptoms recur, patients can simply take another dose of the short-acting medication to treat these symptoms. If rebound becomes a frequent problem, it is better to change to a longer-acting drug, such as one of the dopamine agonists.

It is less common to see rebound with ropinirole (half-life of 6 hours) or pramipexole (half-life of 8 to 12 hours). However, if these drugs are given early enough in the day (before 7 PM) to treat afternoon or evening RLS, they can result in middle-of-the-night rebound symptoms. Longer half-life medications, such as pramipexole ER, ropinirole XL, and cabergoline, long-acting medications such as rotigotine transdermal or off-label treatment with divided doses of short-acting dopamine agonists may alleviate this problem.

■ Augmentation

Augmentation is a worsening of RLS symptoms (**Table 9.5**) caused by the drug that is being used to treat the disorder. For the most part, this problem occurs mainly with drugs that work on the dopamine system, but there have been two articles reporting augmentation with tramadol.[29,30] Usually, the worsening from augmentation occurs weeks or months after initiating therapy for RLS.[31]

The mechanism of augmentation is not yet understood. It may seem strange that a drug that first improves the RLS symptoms later causes a worsening of symptoms. Several theories exist to explain this phenomenon including downregulation of the dopamine receptors (similar to tolerance) and overstimulation of the dopamine D_1 receptors compared with D_2 receptors.[32] It is also thought that iron deficiency may be a key predisposing factor for developing augmentation by causing a reduced function of the dopamine transporter.[32]

Augmentation is Associated With Dopaminergic Drugs

Augmentation of RLS due to L-dopa was first described and studied in 1996,[3] many years after this drug was first used to treat the disorder. This study found that 82% of RLS patients treated with L-dopa developed problems with augmentation. There was an association with dose in that augmentation occurred more readily in those who took ≥200 mg L-dopa per day. Although lower daily doses are less likely to cause augmentation, they still can cause this problem. As augmentation symptoms due to L-dopa tend to be very severe, it is recommended that L-dopa–containing drugs be used only on an intermittent basis.

Augmentation rates appear to be lower with the dopamine agonists.[33] The exact prevalence of augmentation due to dopamine agonists is still not well known. Most of the studies have been performed prior to the development of standardized criteria to diagnose and rate augmentation or have not been structured (usually they are too short) to capture this side effect or have required investigators to volunteer augmentation as a side effect rather than seeking it out specifically. A 2007 study examining the safety of ropinirole found a 2.3% augmentation rate in a 52-week study.[34] However, a 2011 study by Allen[35] using 2003 NIH criteria for diagnosing augmentation (**Figure 9**.7) found the augmentation with the use of ropinirole for an average of 2.7 years was 24%, while a 2012 study[36] using the MPI criteria for augmentation (**Table 9**.5) found a 3% augmentation rate following patients on ropinirole for 66 months.

A 2004 long-term follow-up study found that 32% of those patients on pramipexole developed augmentation[37] while the 2011 study by Allen[35] augmentation rates were 11%. However, a study by Silver[38] that retrospectively looked back at 10 years of RLS treatment in one tertiary clinic found augmentation rates for pramipexole of 7% per year and 5% per year for pergolide. Cabergoline may have a lower rate of augmentation: <3% in one study[39] and 9% in another study.[40] Rates with pergolide vary between 0% and 27%.[41-43] As noted, augmentation rates for rotigotine in the 5-year study using MPI criteria was 13% and in a retrospective study[44] using the MPI criteria to

FIGURE 9.7 — 2003 NIH Criteria for Augmentation Diagnosis

Criterion 1	**Criterion 2** Two or more of the following are present:			
RLS symptoms occur at least 2 h earlier than was typical	Worsening of symptoms after a medication dose increase or symptom improvement after dose decrease	Latency of RLS symptoms at rest is shorter than during the initial course of treatment	The urge to move or sensations are extended to previously unaffected limbs or body parts	The duration of treatment effect is shorter than the duration during the initial therapeutic response	New or worsening of periodic limb movements while awake

Augmented symptoms meeting one of these criteria are present for at least 1 week

Symptoms are present for at least 5 of 7 days

No other medical, psychiatric, behavioral, or pharmacological factors explain the exacerbation of RLS and augmented symptoms

Allen RP, et al. *Sleep Med.* 2011;12(5):431-439

determine augmentation rates found a rate of 8.2% in two double-blind studies and 9.7% in two open-label studies, but no patients discontinued the rotigotine due to this problem.

The lower rates of augmentation with dopamine agonists compared with L-dopa have been attributed to their longer half-life.[41] To date, cabergoline with its >65-hour half-life seems to have the lowest incidence of augmentation. However, the long duration of this drug's action may actually treat augmentation symptoms that occur earlier in the day. Evaluating augmentation may become more difficult as agents with more sustained therapeutic levels are introduced into RLS treatment.

Although lower doses of L-dopa result in fewer problems with augmentation,[3] this has not yet been shown to be the case for dopamine agonists. Despite this, some experts believe that lower doses of a dopamine agonist may help decrease the incidence of augmentation.[32]

It has also been found that augmentation rates are higher in people with a family history of RLS and those who do not have neuropathy associated with their RLS.[45]

Diagnosis and Evaluation

Once the issue of augmentation is understood, most cases should be obvious once the diagnostic criteria (**Figure 9**.7 and **Table 9**.5) are noted. For clinical purposes, either the older 2003 NIH criteria (**Figure 9**.7) or the newer 2007 MPI (**Table 9**.5) should be used, but the older NIH criteria may be simpler to use for physicians. The key to diagnosing augmentation is associating the worsening of symptoms with the initiation of dopamine treatment. This can be particularly difficult when the problem occurs many months or years after the onset of therapy.

Patients will usually complain that after the initial period of weeks, months, or years of experiencing relief from their symptoms with dopamine medication, symptoms begin to occur at least 2 hours earlier in the day. These symptoms may become more intense, may spread to other body parts (especially the arms, but expansion to all other body parts including the face is possible), and the time at rest before symptoms occur may significantly decrease. In addition, the previous dose of medication may not be as effective in decreasing symptoms or last as long. Increasing the dose may help at first, then become less effective and may lead to further augmentation symptoms. Stopping the medication will typically result in a marked increase in symptoms followed by a return to pretreatment levels after a few weeks.

Symptoms must be present for at least 1 week and a minimum of 5 days per week before augmentation can be diagnosed.[33] The onset of symptoms can be as soon as 1 week but typically occurs within 2 months when due to L-dopa[33] and 6 to 9 months[33,37] with dopamine agonists, but can also be delayed by many years with dopamine agonists.

Augmentation must be differentiated from situations that may appear somewhat similar (**Table 9.6**). As RLS tends to worsen slowly with time, one must be sure that the worsening of symptoms is not due to disease progression. This can be difficult at times as the disease may progress in an erratic fashion and the onset of augmentation may be delayed by many years. At times, the only way to decide if augmentation exists is to stop the dopamine drug and see if symptoms revert to where they were prior to treatment (which does not occur with disease progression).

TABLE 9.6 — Differential Diagnosis of Augmentation

- Natural disease progression of RLS
- Rebound
- Tolerance
- Worsening of RLS due to other factors

Initially, rebound may be confused with augmentation in that patients complain about a worsening of symptoms despite therapy. However, rebound occurs at the end of the dose as a late effect while augmentation presents as an earlier onset of symptoms.

Tolerance shares some of the features of augmentation in that the drug effect diminishes; higher doses are needed to treat symptoms and drug responsiveness usually returns after a few weeks off the drug. Due to these similarities, it has been suggested that tolerance may in fact be a subtype of augmentation[37] caused by a similar downregulation of dopamine receptors. However, for diagnostic purposes, tolerance does not result in an earlier onset of RLS symptoms or expansion of symptoms to other body parts.

Worsening of symptoms due to other causes must also be ruled out. Medications (antihistamines, psychiatric medication, etc), iron deficiency, sleep deprivation, alcohol use, and vigorous exercise are among the many different causes that may exacerbate RLS. Before diagnosing augmentation, doctors should search for exacerbating factors. If the worsened RLS symptoms can be linked to one of these extrinsic factors, symptoms may be improved by simply correcting the offending cause.

Treating Augmentation

Although the daily use of L-dopa has decreased considerably so that L-dopa augmentation does not occur as often as in the past, it is still being prescribed on a daily basis in significant quantities. Augmentation that occurs due to L-dopa therapy usually results in very severe RLS symptoms and should be addressed as soon as possible. The medication should be stopped and replacement therapy with a dopamine agonist or other class of medication should be instituted. However, this must be done carefully as RLS symptoms usually dramatically worsen when L-dopa is withdrawn in this setting. Often an opioid may be necessary for breakthrough RLS symptoms until the new therapy reaches therapeutic levels. If a dopamine agonist is used as replacement therapy, it can be titrated up as the L-dopa is weaned down. There is some controversy about replacing one dopaminergic drug with another due to the concern of recurrent augmentation and physicians should be vigilant for its reemergence.

With the decreased use of L-dopa, augmentation with dopamine agonists is now more common in clinical practice. Mild augmentation where symptoms increase mildly and just occur a few hours earlier may be treated by giving the dopamine agonist dose earlier (and possibly increasing the dose modestly) or by giving two split doses with the first dose timed 1 to 2 hours before symptoms. Alternatively, a longer-acting dopamine agonist like the rotigotine patch or even a change to a different short-acting dopamine agonist may be helpful. As described above with L-dopa, replacing one dopaminergic drug with another might cause recurrent augmentation and physicians should be very vigilant for its reemergence. Drug levels should be kept as low as possible and the need for higher doses should alert the physician to the likelihood of worsening augmentation.

Treating severe augmentation is much more difficult and controversial. Many RLS experts believe that the dopamine agonist should be discontinued completely while others suggest that it may be reduced to lower levels. There are no studies evaluating any technique to handle augmentation, so therapy is based on clinical experience. Adding increased doses of dopamine agonists to a patient with severe augmentation (which is what is done by most physicians including specialists who are not RLS experts) will provide temporary relief but will eventually add "fuel to the fire" and cause even worsened symptoms that will perpetuate the vicious cycle of augmentation that demands yet higher doses. Thus, the dopamine agonist must be stopped or decreased.

Whether dopamine agonist doses are abruptly eliminated, tapered off slowly, or reduced to lower levels, RLS symptoms will be dramatically increased over their current worsened state. With no additional treatment, patients may improve (possibly even a marked improvement to minimal or no symptoms) slowly over a few months but the transition period will typically be a hellish experience. Anticonvulsant drugs ($\alpha2\delta$ ligands) may mitigate some of these symptoms but usually are not effective enough for this situation.

Most patients will need a potent opioid (methadone, oxycodone) to treat the dramatically worsened RLS symptoms created by the withdrawal of their dopamine agonist. Physicians who are unwilling or unable to prescribe potent opioids for these patients when other options fail should refer them to another physician. The opioid may need to be prescribed up to three times daily to cover the around-the-clock RLS symptoms that ensue upon reducing or withdrawing dopamine agonists. After a few weeks, the dose of opioids may be gradually reduced as RLS symptoms typically abate somewhat. After a few months, adding an $\alpha2\delta$ ligand may be offered to the patient in order to further reduce or eliminate the need for opioids. Patients may end up on opioid monotherapy, a low dose of an opioid, and an $\alpha2\delta$ ligand, or a low dose of a dopamine agonist, an $\alpha2\delta$ ligand, and an opioid. Treatment should be individualized to the level of RLS symptoms, side effects of treatment, and needs of the patient as is discussed in *Chapter 10*.

Measures that may prevent augmentation from occurring in the first place are keeping the dopamine agonist dose as low as possible, choosing longer-acting dopamine agonists, and keeping serum ferritin levels high (as lower ferritin levels have been associated with increased augmentation[46,47]).

■ Unapproved Dopamine Agonists for Treating RLS

This next group of drugs consists of older dopamine agonists that have been used for RLS and newer ones that are under investigation. The older dopamine agonists may never be FDA approved for RLS due to side effects or because most are already off patent.

It still may be important to be familiar with these drugs as they can be useful at times. The dopamine agonists can be divided into two groups: those that are derived from ergot alkaloids (produced by a fungus that infects rye and other plants) and those that are not related to ergots. Ropinirole, pramipexole, and rotigotine are not derived from ergot alkaloids but most of the other dopamine agonists are in this category (bromocriptine, cabergoline, lisuride, pergolide).

The ergot-derived dopamine agonists all share a common potential adverse effect of fibrosis in the abdomen, lung, and heart.[48] There are many reports of retroperitoneal fibrosis,[49,50] pleuropulmonary fibrosis (interstitial and pleural),[51,52] and cardiac fibrosis (pericardial and valvular).[53-56] In fact, due to the recent finding that the incidence of ergot-induced valvular damage is as high as 22% in one study (cabergoline and pergolide)[57] and 29% with cabergoline and 23% with pergolide in another study,[58] pergolide has been voluntarily removed from the US market. This does not appear to be a problem with the non–ergot-derived dopamine agonists as these same studies found an incidence of either 3% (with no controls)[57] or 0% (6% in controls).[58]

Until further study is done on the problem, ergot-related dopamine agonists (bromocriptine, cabergoline, and pergolide) should be used with caution (and only when all other drugs have failed) with echocardiogram monitoring at regular intervals (3 to 6 months). It is thought that these ergot drugs induce fibrotic changes by activating the $5HT_{2B}$ receptors (a subtype of serotonin receptor) that stimulate fibrocytes. Therefore, ergot drugs, such as lisuride and terguride, that antagonize the $5HT_{2B}$ receptors may not stimulate fibrosis.[59,60] In fact, no reports of fibrotic heart damage have yet appeared for lisuride[61] despite >20 years of clinical use in the same clinical population as other ergot dopamine agonists.

For a convenient reference, these drugs are listed and discussed below alphabetically by generic name, although they differ considerably in the evidence-based rationale for their use in RLS.

Apomorphine

This non–ergot-related drug is a derivative of morphine that has both dopamine agonist and opioid properties and is only approved for use in PD.[62] A few studies have demonstrated its efficacy for RLS in selected cases.[63,64]

Apomorphine is quite different from all of the other dopamine agonists in that it is administered by subcutaneous injection. As such, it is extremely fast acting. This drug should not be given without an antiemetic, as nausea and vomiting are common and significant problems. This drug may be a good choice for postoperative RLS patients who cannot take oral medications and need quick relief from their RLS symptoms.

Bromocriptine

This ergot-derived drug, approved for use in prolactin-producing pituitary tumors and PD, was the first dopamine agonist employed to treat RLS. First described for treating RLS by Sevket Akpinar in 1982,[2] there are only a few studies describing its efficacy for treating RLS.[65-67]

Cabergoline

This is one of the newer ergot-derived dopamine agonist drugs. It is unique in that it has a very long half-life of >65 hours. Studies performed in Europe have demonstrated cabergoline's efficacy and safety for RLS.[68,69]

A benefit of this drug includes its once-daily dosing, which is ideal for patients with severe RLS who otherwise need up to three doses of shorter-acting drugs. In addition, possibly due to its long duration, augmentation rates appear to be quite low. Its side effect profile is similar to that of other dopamine agonists, although one recent study comparing it with L-dopa found that it has a higher incidence of adverse reactions.[70] Like other ergot-derived drugs, it has been implicated in causing fibrosis so it should be used only when there are no other alternatives.

Cabergoline is metabolized in the liver and has an onset of action in about 1 to 3 hours. Dosing is once daily in the evening starting at 0.25 to 0.5 mg and increased on a weekly basis by 0.25 to 0.5 mg, to a maximum dose of 4 mg. The average effective dose for treating RLS is about 2 mg.

Lisuride

This drug, which is not available in the United States, is approved in Europe to treat PD, hyperprolactinemia, and migraine headaches (off label). Lisuride is an ergot-related dopamine agonist. Due to its short half-life and variable bioavailability, this drug is better suited to treat RLS by the transdermal route. Despite its being an ergot-related dopamine drug, it does not appear to cause fibrotic changes, as do the others in this class (see discussion above). There are two open-label studies conducted by the same investigator that showed efficacy and safety in small groups of RLS patients using this drug.[71,72]

Pergolide

This ergot-derived dopamine agonist has recently been voluntarily withdrawn from the US drug market due to its association with fibrotic heart valve damage (see above); as of this writing, it is still available in Europe. Many studies have found it to be an effective treatment for RLS when tolerated.[73-76]

Piribedil

Piribedil is a non–ergot-derived dopamine agonist that is not available in the United States but approved elsewhere for PD, cognitive disorders, and treatment of retinal ischemic manifestations. It is generally prescribed in its slow-release form. There is only one open-label pilot study that examined the use of piribedil in RLS and found it effective in 11 of 13 RLS patients.[77]

Pramipexole ER

This the extended-release form of pramipexole that is available in 0.375 mg, 0.75 mg, 1.5 mg, 2.25 mg, 3 mg, 3.75 mg and 4.5 mg tablets and has been approved only for the treatment of PD. There are no studies published for the use of this 24-hour long-acting drug for treating RLS. However, some RLS specialists prescribe this drug for patients requiring pramipexole two to three times daily due to symptoms starting in the morning. Patients on short-acting pramipexole may be changed over to the equivalent daily dose of pramipexole ER. Patients who are not on a dopamine agonist should be started on the lowest dose and increased to higher doses every 5 to 7 days if needed. However, the concern with using this drug is that all the doses are fairly high and may increase the odds of augmentation occurring despite the long half-life of the drug.

Ropinirole XL

This is the extended-release form of ropinirole that is available in 2 mg, 4 mg, and 8 mg tablets and has been approved only for the treatment of PD. Similar to pramipexole ER above, it is a 24-hour preparation that may be helpful in patients with 24-hour symptoms who might otherwise require three doses of short-acting ropinirole. The concerns with using this drug are similar to that of the extended-release pramipexole.

Terguride

Terguride is a partial dopamine agonist (ergot-derived) that is not available in the United States and is approved to treat hyperprolactinemia. It has a half-life of 4.3 hours and comes to peak concentration in 1 hour.[78] Side effects are similar to those of other dopamine agonists.

Only one open-label study has assessed terguride for treating RLS and found it to be effective in seven RLS patients but not for daytime symptoms.[79]

Anticonvulsants

Anticonvulsant drugs (**Table 9**.7) were the third class of drugs used to treat RLS in modern times (after sedative hypnotics and dopaminergics), with the first report describing carbamazepine in 1983,[80] shortly after the account of L-dopa's use for RLS. Until recently, anticonvulsants were considered second-line drugs.[4] However; this paradigm may be shifting with many RLS experts currently considering the use of the approved $\alpha2\delta$ ligand drugs as equal first-line choices with the dopamine agonists.

TABLE 9.7 — Anticonvulsant Drugs

Anticonvulsant	Individual Dose Range (mg)
Carbamazepine	100-400, up to 3×/day
Gabapentin	100-900, up to 3×/day
Gabapentin enacarbil	300-600 mg once daily
Gabapentin extended release	300-1800 mg/day
Lamotrigine	25-250, up to 2×/day
Levetiracetam	250-1500, up to 2×/day
Oxcarbazepine	150-1200, up to 2×/day
Pregabalin	25-200, up to 3×/day or 75-300, up to 2×/day
Tiagabine	2-16, up to 2×/day
Topiramate	25-200, up to 2×/day
Valproic acid	250-500, up to 2-3×/day
Zonisamide	100-600, once daily

Sedation and dizziness, which may carry over to the next day, tend to be their major limitations. However, when the sedation occurs only at bedtime, it may actually be an advantage when using these drugs. Patients should be advised to take their first dose prior to a day when they do not have to drive so that they can assess whether the drug impairs this function. Suicidal behavior and ideation is a concern with all anticonvulsants and should be discussed with the patient. They may also cause the DRESS syndrome (Drug Reaction with Eosinophilia and Systemic Symptoms) so patients with skin rashes should be monitored closely for the development of systemic symptoms such as fever and checked for eosinophilia.

In addition, anticonvulsants have been suggested to be particularly useful for painful RLS symptoms or for neuropathies that are often associated with RLS. There is currently only one FDA-approved anticonvulsant (gabapentin enacarbil) but there is some evidence-based literature supporting the benefits for other α2δ ligands. The off-label drugs may be used more readily for RLS when patients have comorbid neuropathy or pain for which these drugs have been approved.

The anticonvulsant medications may also relieve anxiety that is a common issue in RLS sufferers. There is a substantial and increasing amount of studies demonstrating the anxiolytic properties of pregabalin[79-83] and one study for gabapentin and tiagabine[84] showing comparable effectiveness with SSRIs and SNRIs.

■ α2δ Ligands

These drugs are structural analogs to GABA but they do not bind to GABA receptors but rather bind to the α2δ subunit of voltage-gated calcium channels in the CNS. The mechanism of their effect on RLS is not clear but these drugs can be very effective for treating RLS symptoms. So far, only gabapentin enacarbil has been approved to treat RLS in the United States.

Gabapentin Enacarbil (Horizant)

This drug was the first non-dopamine agonist drug and only α2δ ligand approved by the FDA (April 2011) for moderate to severe RLS and for postherpetic neuralgia (June 2012). The drug was designed as a prodrug of gabapentin by adding a side-chain to gabapentin. The rational for developing the prodrug is that it takes advantage of the high-capacity solute transporters that are located throughout the small and large intestines. Regular gabapentin uses the low-capacity intestinal transporters that are localized in a small section of the proximal small intestine. As a result, the gabapentin transporters may get easily saturated resulting in a dose-dependent bioavailability; at subtherapeutic doses, 60% of gabapentin is orally bioavailable, but at higher doses its bioavailability is reduced to 35% or less.[85] In addition, the gabapentin transporter has variable rates of expression between individuals.[86] Therefore, as physicians increase the dose of gabapentin when symptoms are inadequately controlled, they will not achieve the proportionally higher levels that they expect and the amount of drug needed will be very unpredictable among patients.

The prodrug gabapentin enacarbil utilizes the high capacity intestinal solute transporters that cannot be saturated at doses well above those used for RLS (300-6000 mg) thus providing dose-proportional bioavailability of about 70%.[87] Furthermore, the gabapentin enacarbil transporters are present throughout the small and large intestine, allowing for the use of a slow-release tablet that releases the drug slowly as the pill transits through the intestines. Once the gabapentin enacarbil is transported through the intestinal wall into the blood stream, it is rapidly hydrolyzed to regular gabapentin and is metabolized similarly to that drug.

It is common for insurance companies and pharmacies to suggest a substitution of regular gabapentin for gabapentin enacarbil stating that they are basically the same drug. However, these drugs are not the same and are not interchangeable. Gabapentin enacarbil has dose-proportional absorption that results in predictable blood levels that are much higher than equivalent doses of regular gabapentin. In addition, due to the slow-release matrix tablets, these blood levels are sustained for much longer times providing a much longer duration of action. Furthermore, gabapentin enacarbil has been studied extensively (see below) for safety and efficacy prior to achieving FDA approval for RLS, while regular gabapentin is not FDA approved for RLS.

There have been several studies confirming the efficacy and safety of gabapentin enacarbil for treating moderate to severe RLS, starting with one by Kushida[88] that was a double-blind 12-week study in 2009 on 222 subjects that demonstrated improved RLS by IRLS and CGI (**Figure 9.8**) and also subjective sleep with 1200 mg daily. Walters (2009) conducted a double-blind, 2-week study with 95 subjects given 600 or 1200 mg once daily which found that only 1200 mg helped participants' RLS symptoms and subjective sleep (more than placebo). Kushida (2009)[89] published another double-blind study (2-week PSG study) on 38 subjects utilizing 1800 mg once daily and found improved RLS and sleep by PSG (decreased stage 1 sleep and increased stage 3 deep sleep).

Bogan (2010)[90] demonstrated that 194 subjects maintained improvement and long-term tolerability for 9 months on 1200 mg in a 24-week single-blind study that followed a 12-week double-blind study extension study. Ellenbogen (2011)[91] published a 52-week open-label extension study after four double-blind studies on 573 subjects. Subjects were given 1200 mg initially but could be adjusted to 600-1800 mg. It is notable that 18% ended up on 600 mg, 52% at 1200 mg, and 30% at 1800 mg. The drug was well tolerated with improvement being sustained for over 4 years (**Figure 9.9**).

Lee published a 12-week double-blind study utilizing 600 mg or 1200 mg in 2012 on 325 subjects that demonstrated that both doses improved RLS and sleep similarly but the side effect of dizziness was significantly more frequent in the 1200-mg group (24%) than the 600-mg group (10%) but sleepiness was similar in both groups (18% in the 1200-mg group and 22% in the 600-mg group).[92] The FDA based its decision to approve only the 600-mg dose partially based upon this study. Winkelman (2011)[93] published a double-blind, placebo-controlled, 4-week, 2-period crossover PSG study on 136 subjects who took 1200 mg and found that side effects were similar to other studies with improved RLS symptoms and decreased PLMAI. The study also showed improvements in sleep maintenance, stage 3 deep sleep, and 75% of the subjects had no

FIGURE 9.8 — Mean (±2 SE) Change From Baseline IRLS Total Score and Investigator-Rated Responders on the CGI-1 by Visit

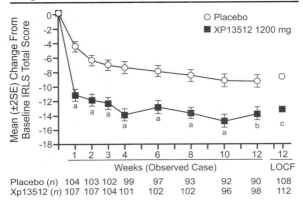

Placebo (n)	104	103	102	99	97	93	92	90	108
Xp13512 (n)	107	107	104	101	102	102	96	98	112

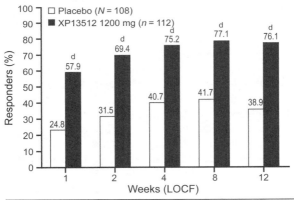

Coprimary end point: adjusted mean treatment difference (week 12, LOC1: -4.0 (analysis of covariance [ANCOVA]: 95% CI: -6.2 to -1.9; $P = 0.0003$) *(top)*. Coprimary end point (week 12, LOCF): OR: 5.1; 95% CI: 2.8 to 9.2; $P < 0.0001$ *(bottom)*.

[a] $P < 0.0001$ vs placebo.
[b] $P = 0.0001$ vs placebo.

Continued

FIGURE 9.8 — *Continued*

[c] $P = 0.0003$ vs placebo; ANCOVA with baseline as covariate and treatment and pooled site as main effects. Unadjusted mean change from baseline at week 12 (LOCF): XP13512 = -13.2; placebo = -8.8.

[d] $P < 0.0001$ vs placebo. Logistic regression adjusted for pooled site. Responders defined as patients with an investigator rating of much improved or very much improved on the CGI-1.

Kushida CA, et al; XP052 Study Group. *Neurology*. 2009;72(5):439-446.

awakenings at all, confirming the positive benefits of this drug on sleep. Inoue (2012)[94] published an open-label, 52-week study on 181 Japanese subjects who took 1200 mg that showed similar results to western studies with improved RLS parameters and side effects of dizziness and sleepiness that occurred mostly in the first month of the study.

The FDA-approved dosing for gabapentin enacarbil for patients with normal renal function is 600 mg taken at 5 to 6 PM with food (food increases the absorption of the drug). A new 300-mg dose has just become available for patients with renal impairment and is dosed based on renal function, as gabapentin is excreted through the kidneys. Patients with creatinine clearances of 30-59 mL/minute should start with 300 mg/day and increase to 600 mg as needed, those with 15 to 29 mL/minute should use 300 mg/day, and those with <15 mL/minute should use 300 mg every other day. The drug is not recommended for patients with renal failure on dialysis.

As noted, gabapentin enacarbil is absorbed in a dose-proportional fashion and rapidly hydrolyzed to regular gabapentin. The drug is then excreted through the kidneys. There are no concerns about significant drug interactions. When taken with food, the drug's T_{max} was 7 hours (hence the rational to take it at 5-6 PM so that sedation peaks at sleep time) and 5 hours when taken on an empty stomach. Absorption is significantly

FIGURE 9.9 — Mean (2 SE) IRLS Total Score by Week and Prior Exposure to Gabapentin Enacarbil (Safety Population)

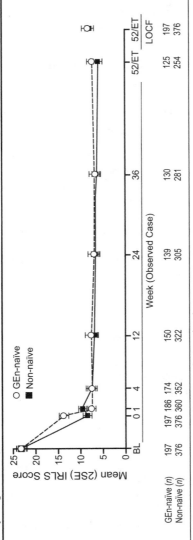

Key: GEn, gabapentin enacarbil; ET, early termination.

Baseline data were obtained at parent study baseline. Week 0 data were obtained at parent study final visit (studies XP052, XP053, and XP081) or visit 3 (study CP083).

Ellenbogen AL, et al. *Clin Neuropharmacol.* 2011;34(1):8-16.

less when taken without food so it may not be effective but it is an alternate method for patients to reduce their dose as they cannot cut the slow-release matrix pill in half. Side effects are similar to other α2δ ligands, with sedation and dizziness being the most common. Other side effects that are shared with other anticonvulsants have been discussed above.

■ Unapproved α2δ Ligands

Gabapentin

Gabapentin was first studied in RLS in 1996 in an open trial of 16 subjects and found to be an effective therapy.[95] Further case studies confirmed its efficacy for both RLS and PLMS in doses between 300 and 1200 mg/day but did not find that it helped sleep parameters (possibly due to only mildly impaired sleep prior to treatment).[96] A subsequent larger and double-blinded study found the drug to be effective for RLS and PLMS and furthermore that sleep parameters (increased total sleep time, sleep efficiency, slow-wave sleep, and decreased stage 1 sleep) were improved at a mean effective dose of 1855 mg/day.[97] That study also found that subjects with increased symptoms of pain benefited the most from gabapentin. This is in keeping with this drug's effect on neuropathic pain.

The two most recent studies compared gabapentin with ropinirole. The first study was an open trial and determined that both drugs are equally effective and well tolerated.[98] However, doses were smaller (300-1200 mg/day) than in other studies and those typically used in practice where sedation often proves troublesome. The second study[99] was a placebo-controlled sleep laboratory trial (40 subjects in a parallel-group design) that compared 300 mg of gabapentin with 0.5 mg of ropinirole and found that only gabapentin improved sleep parameters (subjective sleep, decreased stage 1 sleep, increased slow-wave sleep and REM sleep) while ropinirole decreased PLM (73% decrease) more than gabapentin (35% decrease). Other studies (discussed in *Chapter 11*) have demonstrated its benefit for dialysis patients with RLS.[100,101]

Gabapentin, a structural analogue of γ-aminobutyric acid (GABA) that is an inhibitory neurotransmitter in the central nervous system, is approved in the United States for the treatment of epilepsy and postherpetic neuralgia; however, its mechanism of action is unknown. Side effects include sedation and drowsiness (the most common reasons to discontinue use), dizziness, and peripheral edema. The half-life is about 5 to 7 hours with a T_{max} of 2 to 3 hours and it is eliminated unaltered by the kidneys. While gabapentin is not FDA approved for the treatment of RLS, it is one of the earliest medications studied for RLS treatment.

Typically, gabapentin is started at 300 mg (although 100 mg can be initiated in elderly or sensitive patients), 2 to 3 hours before symptoms usually occur up to three times daily. The dose may be titrated by 100- to 300-mg increments every 3 to 7 days until symptoms are relieved. Although some people are responsive to lower doses of 300 mg, most require 1200 to 2000 mg daily. Dosing can be unpredictable as discussed above due to the non-proportional bioavailability of the drug. Since gabapentin is eliminated unaltered through the kidneys, patients with renal impairment need lower doses and it should be titrated more gradually.

Gabapentin Extended Release (Gralise)

This drug was approved for the once-daily treatment of postherpetic neuralgia in January 2011. It uses a new gastro-retentive technology where the tablet swells in the patient's stomach (especially with a full stomach), which prevents the tablet from traveling through the intestinal tract where gabapentin cannot be absorbed. Absorption usually continues for 10 hours with a T_{max} of 8 hours. Dosing (with the available 300-mg and 600-mg tablets) should start at 300 mg with the evening meal and can be increased, if needed, every few days by 300 mg until symptoms are resolved (to a maximum dose of 1800 mg) or side effects intervene.

This drug has not been studied for treating RLS and is not FDA approved for treating RLS, and there is not much clinical experience available. However, this drug may be helpful for patients with symptoms around-the-clock. However, as it releases regular gabapentin into the intestine, absorption will be dose-dependent and may be erratic. If the pill is not taken with food or if it does not stay in the stomach, absorption may also be dramatically decreased. Side effects are similar to gabapentin.

Pregabalin (Lyrica)

Pregabalin was designed to be a more potent successor to gabapentin. It is approved in the United States for epilepsy, postherpetic neuralgia, and neuropathic pain associated with diabetic peripheral neuropathy. While not FDA approved for the treatment of RLS, pregabalin has been studied for RLS treatment. The first study on pregabalin for RLS was an open-label 2007 trial that found the drug to be effective for 16 of 19 patients with RLS (16 of whom also had a painful neuropathy).[102] Patients were started on 75 mg in the early afternoon and evening then increased or decreased as needed. The average dose was 305 mg and all had satisfactory or good improvement of both RLS and neuropathic pain. This trial was then followed by a 12-week, double-blind, flexible-dose, placebo-controlled 2010 trial[103] with subjects receiving a dose at 9 PM and an additional dose if necessary at 2 PM.

Improvement of the RLS symptoms with pregabalin was found at a mean dose of 322 mg/day (23% of patients needed 450 mg/day). Improvement in PLM was noted with a decrease in stage 1 sleep and an increase in stage 2 and 3 sleep. The typical $\alpha 2\delta$ ligand side effects of sleepiness occurred mostly at doses >450 mg/day. Another 2010 dose ranging study (50, 100, 150, 300, 450 mg/day, or placebo) for 6 weeks,[104] with the dose given 1 to 3 hours before bedtime (subjects had predominately evening symptoms), found the best responses with doses ≥150 mg.

Pregabalin is eliminated primarily by renal excretion and has a half-life of 6 hours and a T_{max} of 1.5

hours (increased to 3 hours with food) and there are no significant drug interactions. The dose of pregabalin should be reduced for patients with renal insufficiency. Side effects are similar to other α2δ ligands, with sedation and dizziness being the most prominent.

■ Other Anticonvulsants

Most of the other anticonvulsants have been used in varying degrees for RLS (**Table 9.7**). They can all be considered second-line agents and all RLS use is off-label. Although there is much less experience with these other drugs, any of them may prove more efficacious or tolerable in given individuals. Therefore, it is often worth trying several in this class until one is found that suits the patient. These medications are also listed alphabetically.

Carbamazepine

As noted,[78] this was the second drug and first anticonvulsant studied for RLS. It has not received too much more attention (except for three studies by the same group[105-107]) as many newer anticonvulsants have since been developed. It is approved in the United States for use in epilepsy and trigeminal neuralgia.

Common side effects include dizziness, drowsiness, unsteadiness, nausea, and vomiting. Rare but severe dermatologic reactions, including toxic epidermal necrolysis and Stevens-Johnson syndrome, may occur as may rare cases of pancytopenia or hepatic failure that require frequent monitoring of blood tests.

The drug is metabolized in the liver and has an initial half-life of 25 to 65 hours, decreasing to 12 to 17 hours with repeated doses. Due to its metabolism by the cytochrome P450 system, it may interact with many other drugs. One study[78] found that doses of 800 to 1000 mg were more effective than lower doses. However, the other studies found improvement compared with placebo using more limited doses of 100 to 300 mg.

Lamotrigine

This drug, [...]
epilepsy and bip[...]
of the phenyltria[...]
existing antiepile[...]
that demonstrated [...]
out of four subjec[...]
dizziness).[108]

Levetiracetam

Levetiracetam [...]
for epilepsy. There i[...]
drug in two patients [...] patients had
RLS symptoms refrac...ry to dopamine agonists, but
responded to 500-1000 mg of levetiracetam at bedtime
and sustained this benefit for >21 months.

Oxcarbazepine

This drug is approved in the United States for
epilepsy. There is only one article discussing the dosing
of oxcarbazepine for RLS; 150 mg twice daily was
used to successfully treat a case of paroxetine-induced
RLS.[110]

Topiramate

Topiramate is approved in the United States for use
in epilepsy and for prophylaxis of migraine headaches.
There has been only one study published on the use of
topiramate in RLS[111] that found it to be an effective
treatment. The mean effective dose was established at
42 mg with a range of 25 to 100 mg.

Valproic Acid

This drug is approved in the United States for use
in epilepsy. At present, only one study has examined
the use of this drug for RLS.[112] This study compared
valproic acid (600 mg) and L-dopa/benserazide
(200/50), using a placebo-controlled, crossover,
double-blind method and found no major difference
between the efficacy of these drugs over a 3-week
test period. However, they found that the decrease in

...LS symptoms was more
...ic acid than with L-dopa.

...ds were the first documented drugs pre-
... for RLS for a woman with RLS whom Sir
...mas Willis effectively treated in 1672. Since Willis'
description and then other successful treatments of
RLS in 1685, several centuries passed before the use
of opioids for RLS was rediscovered. The next known
documentation of the benefit of opioids (except for
Karl Ekbom in 1960[113] and Sevket Akpinar in 1982,[2]
who anecdotally noted that RLS responds to opioids)
occurred in 1984 (2 years after L-dopa and 1 year after
carbamazepine) with the report of three patients who
responded well to treatment with low doses of opioids
(methadone 10 mg or oxycodone 2.5 mg at bedtime).[114]

The often dramatic response of RLS to opioids led
several investigators to speculate that RLS may be in
part due to impairment in the function of the endogenous opiate system.[115,116] The role of the endogenous
opiate system was further investigated with studies
demonstrating that these drugs helped RLS symptoms
and that naloxone could reverse this therapeutic action
but had no effect on its own or after a dopamine agonist.[117-119] Interestingly, the effect of opioids on RLS
may be in part due to their action on the dopaminergic
system as dopamine receptor antagonists block their
therapeutic actions on RLS.[120]

Due to the abuse potential and controlled nature of
these drugs, physicians are often reluctant to use them
to treat RLS especially for long-term treatment of RLS.
However, these drugs are very effective for treating
RLS especially severe, refractory RLS that has not
responded to standard therapy. In a recent 2012 article
giving recommendations for practice guidelines for the
treatment of RLS,[121] the AASM bestowed opioids with
the status of Guideline Treatment (which is the middle
level of their three recommendations between Standard

and Option), indicating that this class of drugs should be prescribed for treating RLS.

■ Wide Variety of Formulations

There are many different opioids available and for the purposes of treating RLS, they are often divided according to their potency into three categories: low, medium, and high (**Table 9.8**). Dosing guidelines vary with the specific drugs (**Table 9.8**). There are very few published data on the use of this class of medication for patients with RLS and none are approved to treat RLS. Some may be prescribed for the approved indications of pain when this occurs as a component of the RLS treatment.

Due to their potential for tolerance and dependence, these drugs are not considered to be a first-line treatment for RLS. However, they can be valuable medications for those who cannot tolerate or do not improve on the dopamine agonists or anticonvulsants. For many severe RLS sufferers, opioids may provide their only source of relief. As these medications tend to onset quickly (usually within 10 to 15 minutes), they are very useful for treating unexpected episodes of RLS on an intermittent basis where there is no risk of tolerance or dependence.

Choosing the correct opioid from the many available may seem difficult, but with an understanding of the drugs, this decision may be easier. Typically, the lowest dose and least potent of these drugs should be tried first, then increased as necessary.

Many of these opioid analgesics are combined with acetaminophen, aspirin, or ibuprofen. Although these additives help reduce pain, they have no therapeutic effect on RLS. Therefore, they can only cause adverse effects without adding any positive benefits and should be avoided when possible. *If possible, opioid analgesics should be chosen in their pure form without any unhelpful (for RLS) additives.*

9

TABLE 9.8 — Opioid Drugs

Drug Name	Usual Dose Range for RLS	Potency for Treating RLS
Codeine	15-60 mg q 4-6 hours	Low
Fentanyl	12.5-25 mcg/hour patch	High
Hydrocodone	2.5-10 mg q 4-6 hours	Medium
Hydromorphone	2-8 mg q 4-6 hours	High
Levorphanol	2-4 mg q 6-8 hours	High
Meperidine, oral	50-300 mg q 3-4 hours	Low
Methadone	5-10 mg q 8 hours	High
Morphine	5-10 mg q 4-6 hours	High
Morphine (controlled-release)	15-30 mg q 12 hours	High
Oxycodone	2.5-10 mg q 4-8 hours	High
Oxycodone (sustained-release)	10-40 q 12 hours	High
Oxymorphone	2.5-5 mg q 4-6 hours	High
Oxymorphone (extended-release)	5-10 mg q 12 hours	High
Pentazocine	50-100 mg q 3-4 hours	Low
Propoxyphene	65-100 mg q 3-4 hours	Low
Tramadol	50-100 mg q 6 hours	Medium
Tramadol (extended-release)	100-300 mg daily	Medium

Side Effects of Opioids

Adverse reactions to opioids tend to be similar and include light-headedness, dizziness, sedation, constipation, nausea, and vomiting. These side effects tend to be dose dependent and are more common among the more potent opioids. Another concern with the more potent opioids is respiratory depression (especially in patients with COPD) and worsening of the very common disorder, sleep apnea (although typically, central sleep apnea is increased with opioids).

Every drug in this class may produce tolerance and dependence when used for chronic therapy. In addition, addiction can occur readily with these drugs in susceptible people (especially in those with a history of substance abuse). Patients should be monitored closely for escalating use of these drugs and carefully managed when this occurs.

■ Low-Potency Opioids

This class includes codeine, meperidine (oral), pentazocine, and propoxyphene. Due to their low potency, these drugs have more leeway than the more potent opioids for causing tolerance and dependence, and they have fewer and less severe side effects. They are very suitable for treating milder RLS symptoms and should be tried before employing the more potent agents.

Codeine

Few studies have evaluated codeine for treating RLS. One study looked retrospectively at people with RLS who used various opioids including codeine (65 to 100 mg) for long-term use.[122] Just as in clinical practice, these investigators found codeine to be effective for long-term use. Another study prospectively administered codeine (30 to 120 mg/day in divided doses) to two subjects who found that the drug improved their RLS symptoms.[117]

Propoxyphene

There are no trials of this drug for RLS patients but the retrospective review noted earlier[122] for codeine also found long-term effectiveness of propoxyphene (65 to 100 mg) for RLS in 25 patients. There is also one case report of a patient who controlled his symptoms with propoxyphene for 5 years[115] and another article that showed benefit prospectively giving the drug (130 to 260 mg/day in divided doses) to three subjects.[117] This drug was withdrawn from the US market in November 2010 due to potentially serious or fatal heart rhythm abnormalities.

■ Medium-Potency Opioids

This class includes the popular drug hydrocodone and the somewhat hard to classify drug tramadol. These drugs are reasonably similar in potency both for pain and RLS management.

Hydrocodone

This opioid has never been studied for treating RLS and no case reports exist for this use. However, as it is a popular drug that most physicians in the United States are quite comfortable using, it is often used to treat RLS symptoms. The problem with using this drug chronically for RLS is that it is always manufactured in combination with a non-narcotic opioid analgesic (acetaminophen, aspirin, or ibuprofen). As such, these additives only increase the risk of side effects without the possibility of benefits for treating RLS. Hydrocodone can be effective in the range of 2.5 mg to 10 mg. For patients who cannot take other opioids, hydrocodone may be purchased in its pure form at a compounding pharmacy but may be fairly expense.

Tramadol

Similar to the opioids, this synthetic opioid-like drug is approved only for the short-term management of acute pain. Although often classified as an opioid, it is considered to be an atypical central-acting opioid-like drug. It is not clear exactly how this drug controls pain as it binds very weakly to the μ-opioid receptors (that are responsible for opioid's antinociceptive effects) and its effects are only partially blocked by naloxone. Its analgesic effects may be due in part from its weak inhibition of the reuptake of norepinephrine and serotonin.[123]

This different action of tramadol may account for its lower potential for abuse.[124-126] For this reason, this drug may be a reasonable choice for treating either pain or RLS. Common side effects include nausea, vomiting, sweating, and dizziness, but these occur much less frequently and less severely than with opioids. This drug is also known to lower the seizure threshold. As noted earlier, recent reports have found that tramadol is the only nondopaminergic drug to cause augmentation.[29,30]

Only one study has examined the use of tramadol for RLS in a long-term (15 to 24 months) open trial.[127] The drug was found to be very effective at 50-150 mg in 10 of 12 subjects.

■ High-Potency Opioids

This class includes the transdermal patch fentanyl, hydromorphone, levorphanol, methadone, morphine, oxycodone, and oxymorphone. *Since this group contains the most potent opioids that have the highest risk of tolerance, dependence, and respiratory depression, they should be prescribed with caution and only by physicians who are very familiar with their use.*

These medications are not considered as drugs of first choice but should be considered in the appropriate circumstances. They are often necessary for refractory RLS patients when dopamine agonists and anticonvulsants fail or for patients with severe RLS symptoms. Patients with augmentation who must stop their dopamine agonist often will not be able to do so without the aid of these potent opioids. Physicians who treat these types of patients and are unable or unwilling to prescribe potent opioids should refer them to another physician who can treat them appropriately.

With proper patient selection (avoid patients with a history of drug abuse) and careful monitoring of patients' dosage and drug use, these medications are both effective and reasonably safe. Tolerance and dependence should occur infrequently and these drugs should not be withheld due to their stigma as dangerous and addicting narcotics. Patients typically do not escalate their doses rapidly and tend to remain stable in their opioid-dose levels with little change with use for a decade or longer (see below).

Fentanyl Transdermal Patches

This potent opioid, which is approved in the United States only for use in chronic pain, has the unique delivery system of a transdermal patch. There are currently no studies or reports on this drug for its use in RLS. Some specialists prescribe this drug for an occasional case of severe RLS that occurs around the clock and needs continuous treatment.

Fentanyl should be started at its lowest dose of 12.5 mcg/hour (one patch every 3 days), and increased after 6 days to 25 mcg/hour, if necessary.

Hydromorphone, Levorphanol, and Oxymorphone

There are no studies or case reports on these three very potent opioids that are approved in the United States only for relief of moderate to severe pain. There is little experience with these medications for RLS; however, some physicians who are familiar with them have found that they are quite effective at relieving RLS symptoms. Since oxymorphone has been released only more recently in the United States in its oral form, experience with this drug for any purpose is minimal. Suggested doses for these drugs are detailed in **Table 9.8**.

Methadone

This drug is approved for treating severe pain and for narcotic addiction detoxification and maintenance. Several reports found this drug to be beneficial for treating RLS. One study describes a patient who benefited from 10 mg at bedtime and worsened when the dose was reduced.[114] Another study prospectively gave methadone (5-20 mg/day, usually in two divided doses) to two subjects and found it to be effective.[117] Eight further patients benefiting from the long-term use of methadone 10 mg were noted in a retrospective review.[122] A 2005 study by Ondo retrospectively reviewed 29 patients in whom dopaminergic therapy failed; they then took methadone (average dose was 16 mg/day and range was 5-40 mg/day, usually in two equal doses) and found that 17 of them remained on the drug with marked reduction in their RLS symptoms for an average of 23 months.[128] Adverse events were mild to moderate and similar to those seen with opioids in general; no subjects developed tolerance.

A 2011 study[129] that retrospectively examined the use of methadone in a tertiary RLS clinic found that after 15% of RLS patients started on methadone stopped the drug in the first year (due to side effects), no patients discontinued the drug for the subsequent 9 years of follow-up. This is in stark contrast to pramipexole and pergolide that had dropout rates after the first year of 9% and 8% per year, respectively, over the subsequent 9 years (mostly due to augmentation). Furthermore, the methadone median dose at 6 months was 10 mg and was no more than 10 mg greater at 8 to 10 years of treatment. This is similar to the 23-month duration study above by Ondo (2005)[128] that found starting average methadone doses at 13 mg/day compared with 16 mg/day at the end of the study.

Despite the lack of proper medical studies to determine the efficacy, safety, and dosing of this drug, there is a significant cadre of RLS specialists who preferentially use methadone over other opioids to treat refractory or severe RLS cases. This is due to several properties of methadone that make it useful for managing RLS. Furthermore, this drug tends to be more effective for RLS and better tolerated than other opioids for the majority of RLS patients (based on clinical experience).

Due to its long half-life, methadone can relieve pain for 8 to 12 hours.[130] Similarly, it tends to eliminate RLS symptoms longer than most drugs, allowing for two to three doses per day to be effective. Its use for narcotic addiction supports its decreased abuse potential compared with other opioids.[131] Methadone may cause less tolerance than other opioids as it does not cause intracellular forskolin-stimulated cAMP accumulation, a mechanism thought to contribute to opioid tolerance.[132] Clinical experience also supports the low level of tolerance to this drug with only mild increases in dose over many years of treatment and rare cases of rapid dose escalation (as long as patients are selected properly and monitored appropriately).

Morphine

This drug is approved in the United States only for the treatment of moderate to severe pain. It is not commonly employed for treating RLS; however, there are two articles that report using it for RLS.[133,134]

Oxycodone

This drug is approved in the United States only for the treatment of moderate to severe pain. A few studies have been done to evaluate the treatment of RLS with oxycodone. The first study reports two cases that responded very well to oxycodone at 2.5 mg.[114] The next study retrospectively reviewed 30 patients who did well with 5 mg oxycodone for long-term therapy.[122] The last study, which is a double-blind, placebo, cross-over protocol, demonstrated that flexible dosing of oxycodone 5-25 mg/day (taken in two to three divided doses) significantly improved all RLS symptoms.[135] The average dose was between 10 and 15 mg/day.

When patients have adverse reactions to methadone, this is often the next opioid chosen by many RLS experts. More frequent dosing is often necessary as the drug has a relatively short duration of action of about 4 to 6 hours. For patients who need three or more tablets per day, switching to the 12-hour long-acting oxycodone preparation may be helpful.

Sedative Hypnotics

Although these drugs were among the first used and reported on (in 1979) for treating RLS,[136] there is considerable controversy about whether they actually relieve RLS symptoms. Most RLS experts use these drugs sparingly to treat RLS symptoms, for which they are not approved, but rather to treat the insomnia associated with RLS (for which many of them are approved).

The early studies that were mostly open-label protocols reported dramatic improvements with these drugs (eg, clonazepam). Sleep disruption is the major complaint of RLS sufferers[137] and the sedative-hypnotic drugs address this problem extremely well. It is not entirely clear from these early reports whether the RLS symptoms were more bedtime related or were also prominent earlier in the day and whether the daytime symptoms were equally relieved.

The second concern when assessing the open-label studies is the strong placebo effect in RLS studies. This placebo effect may account for much of the relief of any daytime symptoms attributed to the benzodiazepines. Even in the placebo-controlled trials, the marked improvement of disruptive sleep patterns due to the use of these drugs and resultant increased daytime well-being may decrease the perception of bothersome daytime RLS symptoms.

Another concern about the use of sedative hypnotics (especially with their daytime use or with the bedtime use of long-acting ones that may spill over into the next day) is that they have a potential for worsening daytime RLS symptoms and increasing the risk of accidents from activities that require vigilance. It is well accepted that RLS symptoms increase with both physical and mental rest[137] so that drugs that cause sedation may actually increase RLS symptoms. One study found that intravenous administration of diphenhydramine 25 mg or lorazepam 0.5 mg to 12 RLS patients who were adequately treated with dopamine agonists caused both similar and severe exacerbation of their otherwise controlled RLS symptoms.[138]

However, the real goal of physicians is to make patients feel better. If these drugs do accomplish this goal for RLS sufferers, they should be considered, especially when other drugs have not been helpful. Furthermore, a significant group of RLS sufferers do state that the sedative-hypnotic drugs relieve their symptoms. Additionally, these drugs markedly decrease awakenings and stage 1 sleep from PLM,[139] which are so common in RLS sufferers, which may be another benefit from their use (see *Chapter 11*).

It is not uncommon for long-time RLS sufferers to have continued insomnia even after their symptoms have been resolved by treatment. After years of not sleeping well, they typically develop a conditioned insomnia. The use of sedative-hypnotic drugs may be invaluable to break this poor sleep cycle.

However, when choosing a sedative hypnotic, it is generally best to select one that has a quick onset to promote sleep initiation and a relatively short half-life to prevent daytime sleepiness or drowsiness that in turn may promote increased RLS symptoms (**Table 9.9**). For chronic daily use, the nonbenzodiazepines (**Table 9.10**) are far more preferred due to their decreased side effect profile and markedly decreased risk of tolerance and dependence.

■ Benzodiazepines

This group comprises several drugs that share similarities and are marketed either as hypnotics for inducing sleep or to treat anxiety (**Table 9.9**). Despite being approved and marketed only as sedatives, some of these drugs may be suitable for use as hypnotics. The following discussion will review the literature on the use of these medications for treating RLS. Drugs are listed alphabetically.

Alprazolam

An open-label study examined alprazolam at 0.5 mg to 1 mg at bedtime in 10 subjects with RLS.[140]

TABLE 9.9 — Benzodiazepines (Hypnotics and Sedatives)

Generic Drug Name	Half-Life (hours)	Individual Dose Range (mg)	Approved as a Hypnotic for Sleep
Alprazolam	6-12	0.25-1	No
Clonazepam	30-40	0.5-2	No
Clorazepate	48	7.5-30	No
Chlordiazepoxide	7-48	2-25	No
Diazepam	24-100	2-10	No
Estazolam	10-24	0.5-2	Yes
Flurazepam	47-100	15-30	Yes
Lorazepam	10-20	0.5-2	No
Oxazapam	8	10-30	No
Quazepam	39-73	7.5-30	Yes
Temazepam	9.5-12.5	7.5-30	Yes
Triazolam	1.5-5.5	0.125-0.5	Yes

9

TABLE 9.10 — Nonbenzodiazepine Hypnotics

Generic Drug Name	Half-Life (hours)	Individual Dose Range (mg)
Ramelteon	1-2.6	8
Eszopiclone	6	1-3
Zaleplon	1	10-20
Zolpidem	2.5	2.5-10
Zolpidem (slow-release)	2.8	6.25-12.5

They found that eight of their 10 patients improved on the alprazolam. One patient stated that taking 0.5 mg of the drug before going to the theater provided her with relief throughout the entire evening.

Clonazepam

The first report on the use of this drug for RLS was a letter to the editor in 1979 that described two people who benefited greatly from the bedtime and evening use of clonazepam 0.5-1 mg.[136] This was followed by another letter to the editor that reported on three more people who benefited from taking clonazepam 0.5 mg one to three times daily.[141] The first double-blind crossover trial of clonazepam in RLS found it to be more effective on six subjects compared with placebo and quite safe to use.[142] They also examined the use of vibration to the leg and did not find it significantly effective.

However, the next study, also a placebo-controlled, double-blind, crossover study, did not find clonazepam to be more effective than placebo on six subjects.[143] This article clearly adds to the controversy about whether clonazepam relieves RLS symptoms or merely helps RLS patients sleep better.

Clonazepam is a readily available and inexpensive drug and as such has a particular physician following for treating RLS. As noted, it clearly resolves the insomnia associated with RLS and improves well-being in people who are suffering prior to treatment.

The concern with this drug is that it has a 30 to 40 hour half-life, which may easily result in next-day sedation, especially when taken for several nights consecutively. This daytime sedation is often not apparent to the patient especially when compared with their previous RLS-induced sleep-deprived state. As other shorter-acting sedative hypnotics have been shown to be effective for RLS (see below), there are alternatives that may be safer and inexpensive.

In addition, clonazepam, like other benzodiazepines, may cause tolerance and dependence when used on a daily basis. Using nonbenzodiazepines dramatically diminishes this risk.

Temazepam

No studies have yet evaluated this drug for RLS. However, one study showed the efficacy of temazepam for PLM.[100]

Triazolam

There is one report of triazolam 0.25 mg taken at bedtime helping one patient with RLS for 6 months.[144] This patient stopped the drug and experienced recurrence of her symptoms within 48 hours.

There are two articles demonstrating the benefits of triazolam for PLM.[145,146] These studies have demonstrated improvements in sleep architecture by increasing total sleep time, decreasing the number of awakenings and arousals, decreasing stage 1 sleep while increasing stage 2 sleep, and increasing sleep efficiency. Additionally, daytime sleepiness was diminished. Triazolam did not decrease the PLM, but it did markedly decrease the arousals and awakenings from the PLM.

Triazolam has a quick onset of action and a short half-life of 1.5 to 5.5 hours that limits next-day drowsiness. Unfortunately, this drug has been associated with a significant degree of retrograde amnesia and rebound insomnia.

■ Nonbenzodiazepines

Most sleep specialists prefer using this class of drugs for treating insomnia. They have a short half-life and are associated with a limited degree of dependence or tolerance. There is only one study for RLS with zolpidem, which is discussed below. However, any of these drugs may be beneficial to help patients fall asleep, whether or not the insomnia is due to RLS symptoms.

Eszopiclone and Zaleplon

These two drugs fill some of the gaps that are not fully covered by zolpidem therapy as zaleplon has a very short half-life of 1 hour while eszopiclone has a half-life of 6 hours compared with the 2.5 hours for zolpidem. Although there are no studies of these drugs for RLS, it is likely that they may work fairly similarly to zolpidem.

Ramelteon

This drug is different from all of the other hypnotic drugs discussed. It does not act upon the GABA receptors that help promote sleep but rather on the melatonin receptors. This drug, which has relatively few side effects, is indicated for sleep-onset insomnia, since its effects on improving sleep maintenance are much less pronounced.[147]

Zolpidem

This drug was studied for RLS in one open-label prospective trial on eight subjects who were unresponsive to or could not tolerate L-dopa and benzodiazepines.[148] The researchers found that all patients had complete relief from their RLS symptoms within an average of 4 days of starting zolpidem 10 mg that lasted 12 to 30 months with no relapses or side effects.

Zolpidem has a quick onset of action and a short half-life of 2.5 hours. It has been associated with abnormal sleep-related behaviors, such as sleep-walking, sleep-talking, or a sleep-related eating disorder,[149] but otherwise has been well tolerated. There is a controlled-release version of this drug that increases the half-life to 2.8 hours and may act as long as eszopiclone and a smaller dosage sublingual tablet (1.75 mg and 3.5 mg) that may approximate the effect of zaleplon and should be helpful for middle of the night awakenings.

Other Pharmacologic Options

These other drugs do not fit into the four major categories of drugs that are commonly used to treat RLS. At present, there is little empirical evidence or experience to support the use of these agents, and none are FDA approved for therapy of RLS. However, in cases where the standard drugs are not effective or tolerated, RLS specialists have considered them. They include: amantadine,[150] botulinum toxin type-A,[151] clonidine,[152-157] and propranolol.[158-162]

Vitamins and minerals have also been suggested for RLS therapy. These include: vitamin B_{12}[163,164] vitamin E,[165,166] folic acid,[163,164,167,168] and magnesium.[169-171] However, further evidence is necessary before these supplements can be recommended for treating RLS.

9

REFERENCES

1. Aurora RN, Kristo DA, Bista SR, Rowley JA, Zak RS, Casey KR, et al. The treatement of restless legs syndrome and periodic limb movement disorder in adults – an update for 2012: Practice parameters with an evidence-based systematic review and meta-analyses. *Sleep*. 2012;35:1039-1062.

2. Akpinar S. Treatment of restless legs syndrome with levodopa plus benserazide. *Arch Neurol*. 1982;39:739.

3. Allen RP, Earley CJ. Augmentation of the restless legs syndrome with carbidopa/levodopa. *Sleep*. 1996;19:205-213.

4. Silber MH, Ehrenberg BL, Allen RP, et al; Medical Advisory Board of the Restless Legs Syndrome Foundation. An algorithm for the management of restless legs syndrome. *Mayo Clin Proc*. 2004;79:916-922.

5. Silber MH, Girish M, Izurieta R. Pramipexole in the management of restless legs syndrome: an extended study. *Sleep*. 2003; 26:819-821.

6. Partinen M, Hirvonen K, Jama L, et al. Efficacy and safety of pramipexole in idiopathic restless legs syndrome: a polysomnographic dose-finding study—the PRELUDE study. *Sleep Med*. 2006;7:407-417.

7. Trenkwalder C, Stiasny-Kolster K, Kupsch A, Oertel WH, Koester J, Reess J. Controlled withdrawal of pramipexole after 6 months of open-label treatment in patients with restless legs syndrome. *Mov Disord*. 2006;21:1404-1410.

8. Winkelman JW, Sethi KD, Kushida CA, et al. Efficacy and safety of pramipexole in restless legs syndrome. *Neurology*. 2006;67:1034-1039.

9. Montplaisir J, Fantini ML, Desautels A, Michaud M, Petit D, Filipini D. Long-term treatment with pramipexole in restless legs syndrome. *Eur J Neurol*. 2006;13:1306-1311.

10. Oertel WH, Stiasny-Kolster K, Bergtholdt B, et al. Pramipexole RLS Study Group. Efficacy of pramipexole in restless legs syndrome: a six-week, multicenter, randomized, double-blind study (effect-RLS study). *Mov Disord*. 2007;22:213-219.

11. Trenkwalder C, Garcia-Borreguero D, Montagna P, et al. Therapy with Ropiunirole; Efficacy and Tolerability in RLS 1 Study Group. Ropinirole in the treatment of restless legs syndrome: results from the TREAT RLS 1 study, a 12 week, randomised, placebo controlled study in 10 European countries. *J Neurol Neurosurg Psychiatry*. 2004;75:92-97.

12. Walters AS, Ondo WG, Dreykluft T, Grunstein R, Lee D, Sethi K; TREAT RLS 2 (Therapy with Ropinirole: Efficacy And Tolerability in RLS 2) Study Group. Ropinirole is effective in the treatment of restless legs syndrome. TREAT RLS 2: a 12-week, double-blind, randomized, parallel-group, placebo-controlled study. *Mov Disord*. 2004;19:1414-1423.

13. Allen R, Becker PM, Bogan R, et al. Ropinirole decreases periodic leg movements and improves sleep parameters in patients with restless legs syndrome. *Sleep*. 2004;27:907-914.

14. Bogan RK, Fry JM, Schmidt MH, Carson SW, Ritchie SY; TREAT RLS US Study Group. Ropinirole in the treatment of patients with restless legs syndrome: a US-based randomized, double-blind, placebo-controlled clinical trial. *Mayo Clin Proc*. 2006;81:17-27.

15. Stiasny-Kolster K, Kohnen R, Schollmayer E, Moller JC, Oertel WH; Rotigotine Sp 666 Study Group. Patch application of the dopamine agonist rotigotine to patients with moderate to advanced stages of restless legs syndrome: a double-blind, placebo-controlled pilot study. *Mov Disord*. 2004;19:1432-1438.

16. Oertel WH, Benes H, Garcia-Borreguero D; On behalf of the Rotigotine SP 709 Study Group. Efficacy of rotigotine transdermal system in severe restless legs syndrome: A randomized, double-blind, placebo-controlled, six-week dose-finding trial in Europe. *Sleep Med*. 2008;9:3:228-239.

17. Trenkwalder C, Benes H, Poewe W, et al. Efficacy of rotigotine for treatment of moderate-to-severe restless legs syndrome: a randomised, double-blind, placebo-controlled trial. *Lancet Neurol*. 2008;7(7):595-604.

18. Hening WA, Allen RP, Ondo WG. Rotigotine improves restless legs syndrome: a 6-month randomized, double-blind, placebo-controlled trial in the United States. *Mov Disord*. 2010; 25(11):1675-1683.

19. Schreglmann SR, Gantenbein AR, Eisele G, Baumann CR. Parkinsonism Transdermal rotigotine causes impulse control disorders in patients with restless legs syndrome. *Relat Disord*. 2012;18(2):207-209.

20. Dodd ML, Klos KJ, Bower JH, Geda YE, Josephs KA, Ahlskog JE. Pathological gambling caused by drugs used to treat Parkinson disease. *Arch Neurol*. 2005;62:1377-1381.

21. Nirenberg MJ, Waters C. Compulsive eating and weight gain related to dopamine agonist use. *Mov Disord*. 2006;21:524-529.

9

22. Weintraub D, Siderowf AD, Potenza MN, et al. Association of dopamine agonist use with impulse control disorders in Parkinson disease. *Arch Neurol.* 2006;63:969-973.

23. Tippmann-Peikert M, Park JG, Boeve BF, Shepard JW, Silber MH. Pathologic gambling in patients with restless legs syndrome treated with dopaminergic agonists. *Neurology.* 2007; 68:301-303.

24. Quickfall J, Suchowersky O. Pathological gambling associated with dopamine agonist use in restless legs syndrome. *Parkinsonism Relat Disord.* 2007;13(8):535-536.

25. Driver-Dunckley ED, Noble BN, Hentz JG, et al. Gambling and increased sexual desire with dopaminergic medications in restless legs syndrome. *Clin Neuropharmacol.* 2007;30(5):249-155.

26. Cornelius JR, Tippmann-Peikert M, Slocumb NL, Frerichs CF, Silber MH. Impulse control disorders with the use of dopaminergic agents in restless legs syndrome: a case-control study. *Sleep.* 2010;33(1):81-87.

27. Ondo WG, Lai D. Predictors of impulsivity and reward seeking behavior with dopamine agonists. *Parkinsonism Relat Disord.* 2008;14(1):28-32.

28. Guilleminault C, Cetel M, Philip P. Dopaminergic treatment of restless legs and rebound phenomenon. *Neurology.* 1993;43:445.

29. Earley CJ, Allen RP. Restless legs syndrome augmentation associated with tramadol. *Sleep Med.* 2006;7:592-593.

30. Vetrugno R, La Morgia C, D'Angelo R, et al. Augmentation of restless legs syndrome with long-term tramadol treatment. *Mov Disord.* 2007;22:424-427.

31. Garcia-Borreguero D, Allen RP, Kohnen R, et al; International Restless Legs Syndrome Study Group. Diagnostic standards for dopaminergic augmentation of restless legs syndrome: report from a World Association of Sleep Medicine–International Restless Legs Syndrome Study Group consensus conference at the Max Planck Institute. *Sleep Med.* 2007;8(5):520-530.

32. Paulus W, Trenkwalder C. Less is more: pathophysiology of dopaminergic-therapy-related augmentation in restless legs syndrome. *Lancet Neurol.* 2006;5:878-886.

33. Allen RP, Picchietti D, Hening WA, Trenkwalder C, Walters AS, Montplaisi J; Restless Legs Syndrome Diagnosis and Epidemiology workshop at the National Institutes of Health; International Restless Legs Syndrome Study Group. Restless legs syndrome: diagnostic criteria, special considerations, and

epidemiology. A report from the restless legs syndrome diagnosis and epidemiology workshop at the National Institutes of Health. *Sleep Med.* 2003;4:101-119.

34. Garcia-Borreguero D, Grunstein R, Sridhar G, et al. A 52-week open-label study of the long-term safety of ropinirole in patients with restless legs syndrome. *Sleep Med.* 2007;8(7-8):742-752.

35. Allen RP, Ondo WG, Ball E. et al. Restless legs syndrome (RLS) augmentation associated with dopamine agonist and levodopa usage in a community sample. *Sleep Med.* 2011; 12(5):431-439.

36. García-Borreguero D, Högl B, Ferini-Strambi L, et al. Systematic evaluation of augmentation during treatment with ropinirole in restless legs syndrome (Willis-Ekbom disease): results from a prospective, multicenter study over 66 weeks. *Mov Disord.* 2012;27(2):277-283.

37. Winkelman JW, Johnston L. Augmentation and tolerance with long-term pramipexole treatment of restless legs syndrome (RLS). *Sleep Med.* 2004;5:9-14.

38. Silver N, Allen RP, Senerth J, Earley CJ. A 10-year, longitudinal assessment of dopamine agonists and methadone in the treatment of restless legs syndrome. *Sleep Med.* 2011; 12(5):440-444.

39. Benes H, Heinrich CR, Ueberall MA, Kohnen R. Long-term safety and efficacy of cabergoline for the treatment of idiopathic restless legs syndrome: results from an open-label 6-month clinical trial. *Sleep.* 2004;27:674-682.

40. Stiasny-Kolster K, Benes H, Peglau I, et al. Effective cabergoline treatment in idiopathic restless legs syndrome. *Neurology.* 2004;63:2272-2279.

41. Silber MH, Shepard JW Jr, Wisbey JA. Pergolide in the management of restless legs syndrome: an extended study. *Sleep.* 1997;20:878-882.

42. Winkelmann J, Wetter TC, Stiasny K, Oertel WH, Trenkwalder C. Treatment of restless leg syndrome with pergolide--an open clinical trial. *Mov Disord.* 1998;13:566-569.

43. Earley CJ, Yaffee JB, Allen RP. Randomized, double-blind, placebo-controlled trial of pergolide in restless legs syndrome. *Neurology.* 1998;51:1599-1602.

44. Beneš H, García-Borreguero D, Ferini-Strambi L, Schollmayer E, Fichtner A, Kohnen R. Augmentation in the treatment of restless legs syndrome with transdermal rotigotine. *Sleep Med.* 2012;13(6):589-597.

9

45. Ondo W, Romanyshyn J, Vuong KD, Lai D. Long-term treatment of restless legs syndrome with dopamine agonists. *Arch Neurol*. 2004;61:1393-1397.

46. Trenkwalder C, Högl B, Benes H, Kohnen R. Augmentation in restless legs syndrome is associated with low ferritin. *Sleep Med*. 2008;9(5):572-574.

47. Frauscher B, Gschliesser V, Brandauer E, et al. The severity range of restless legs syndrome (RLS) and augmentation in a prospective patient cohort: association with ferritin levels. *Sleep Med*. 2009;10(6):611-615.

48. Kvernmo T, Hartter S, Burger E. A review of the receptor-binding and pharmacokinetic properties of dopamine agonists. *Clin Ther*. 2006;28:1065-1078.

49. Kains JP, Hardy JC, Chevalier C, Collier A. Retroperitoneal fibrosis in two patients with Parkinson's disease treated with bromocriptine. *Acta Clin Belg*. 1990;45:306-310.

50. Sanchez-Chapado M, Angulo Cuesta J, Guil Cid M, Jimenez FJ, Lopez Alvarez YJ. Retroperitoneal fibrosis secondary to treatment with L-dopa analogues for Parkinson disease. *Arch Esp Urol*. 1995;48:979-983.

51. Danoff SK, Grasso ME, Terry PB, Flynn JA. Pleuropulmonary disease due to pergolide use for restless legs syndrome. *Chest*. 2001;120:313-316.

52. Townsend M, MacIver DH. Constrictive pericarditis and pleuropulmonary fibrosis secondary to cabergoline treatment for Parkinson's disease. *Heart*. 2004;90:e47.

53. Champagne S, Coste E, Peyriere H, et al. Chronic constrictive pericarditis induced by long-term bromocriptine therapy: report of two cases. *Ann Pharmacother*. 1999;33:1050-1054.

54. Serratrice J, Disdier P, Habib G, Viallet F, Weiller PJ. Fibrotic valvular heart disease subsequent to bromocriptine treatment. *Cardiol Rev*. 2002;10:334-336.

55. Balachandran KP, Stewart D, Berg GA, Oldroyd KG. Chronic pericardial constriction linked to the antiparkinsonian dopamine agonist pergolide. *Postgrad Med J*. 2002;78:49-50.

56. Horvath J, Fross RD, Kleiner-Fisman G, et al. Severe multivalvular heart disease: a new complication of the ergot derivative dopamine agonists. *Mov Disord*. 2004;19:656-662.

57. Junghanns S, Fuhrmann JT, Simonis G, et al. Valvular heart disease in Parkinson's disease patients treated with dopamine agonists: a reader-blinded monocenter echocardiography study. *Mov Disord*. 2007;22:234-238.

58. Zanettini R, Antonini A, Gatto G, Gentile R, Tesei S, Pezzoli G. Valvular heart disease and the use of dopamine agonists for Parkinson's disease. *N Engl J Med*. 2007;356:39-46.

59. Horowski R, Jahnichen S, Pertz HH. Fibrotic valvular heart disease is not related to chemical class but to biological function: 5-HT2B receptor activation plays crucial role. *Mov Disord*. 2004;19:1523-1524.

60. Jahnichen S, Horowski R, Pertz HH. Agonism at 5-HT2B receptors is not a class effect of the ergolines. *Eur J Pharmacol*. 2005;513:225-228.

61. Hofmann C, Penner U, Dorow R, et al. Lisuride, a dopamine receptor agonist with 5-HT2B receptor antagonist properties: absence of cardiac valvulopathy adverse drug reaction reports supports the concept of a crucial role for 5-HT2B receptor agonism in cardiac valvular fibrosis. *Clin Neuropharmacol*. 2006;29:80-86.

62. Tribl GG, Sycha T, Kotzailias N, Zeitlhofer J, Auff E. Apomorphine in idiopathic restless legs syndrome: an exploratory study. *J Neurol Neurosurg Psychiatry*. 2005;76:181-185.

63. Reuter I, Ellis CM, Ray Chaudhuri K. Nocturnal subcutaneous apomorphine infusion in Parkinson's disease and restless legs syndrome. *Acta Neurol Scand*. 1999;100:163-167.

64. Tings T, Stiens G, Paulus W, Trenkwalder C, Happe S. Treatment of restless legs syndrome with subcutaneous apomorphine in a patient with short bowel syndrome. *J Neurol*. 2005;252:361-363.

65. Akpinar S. Restless legs syndrome treatment with dopaminergic drugs. *Clin Neuropharmacol*. 1987;10:69-79.

66. Walters AS, Hening WA, Kavey N, Chokroverty S, Gidro-Frank S. A double-blind randomized crossover trial of bromocriptine and placebo in restless legs syndrome. *Ann Neurol*. 1988;24:455-458.

67. Becker PM, Jamieson AO, Brown WD. Dopaminergic agents in restless legs syndrome and periodic limb movements of sleep: response and complications of extended treatment in 49 cases. *Sleep*. 1993;16:713-716.

68. Benes H, Heinrich CR, Ueberall MA, Kohnen R. Long-term safety and efficacy of cabergoline for the treatment of idiopathic restless legs syndrome: results from an open-label 6-month clinical trial. *Sleep*. 2004;27:674-682.

69. Stiasny-Kolster K, Benes H, Peglau I, et al. Effective cabergoline treatment in idiopathic restless legs syndrome. *Neurology*. 2004;63:2272-2279.

9

70. Trenkwalder C, Benes H, Grote L, et al; CALDIR Study Group. Cabergoline compared to levodopa in the treatment of patients with severe restless legs syndrome: results from a multi-center, randomized, active controlled trial. *Mov Disord.* 2007;22:696-703.

71. Benes H. Transdermal lisuride: short-term efficacy and tolerability study in patients with severe restless legs syndrome. *Sleep Med.* 2006;7:31-35.

72. Benes H, Deissler A, Rodenbeck A, Engfer A, Kohnen R. Lisuride treatment of restless legs syndrome: first studies with monotherapy in de novo patients and in combination with levodopa in advanced disease. *J Neural Transm.* 2006;113:87-92.

73. Silber MH, Shepard JW Jr, Wisbey JA. Pergolide in the management of restless legs syndrome: an extended study. *Sleep.* 1997;20:878-882.

74. Earley CJ, Yaffee JB, Allen RP. Randomized, double-blind, placebo-controlled trial of pergolide in restless legs syndrome. *Neurology.* 1998;51:1599-1602.

75. Stiasny K, Wetter TC, Winkelmann J, et al. Long-term effects of pergolide in the treatment of restless legs syndrome. *Neurology.* 2001;56:1399-1402.

76. Trenkwalder C, Hundemer HP, Lledo A, et al; PEARLS Study Group. Efficacy of pergolide in treatment of restless legs syndrome: the PEARLS Study. *Neurology.* 2004;62:1391-1397.

77. Evidente VG. Piribedil for restless legs syndrome: a pilot study. *Mov Disord.* 2001;16:579-581.

78. Lundvall O, Abom PE, Holm R. Carbamazepine in restless legs. A controlled pilot study. *Eur J Clin Pharmacol.* 1983;25:323-324.

79. Feltner DE, Crockatt JG, Dubovsky SJ, et al. A randomized, double-blind, placebo-controlled, fixed-dose, multicenter study of pregabalin in patients with generalized anxiety disorder. *J Clin Psychopharmacol.* 2003;23(3):240-249.

80. Montgomery SA, Tobias K, Zornberg GL, Kasper S, Pande AC. Efficacy and safety of pregabalin in the treatment of generalized anxiety disorder: a 6-week, multicenter, randomized, double-blind, placebo-controlled comparison of pregabalin and venlafaxine. *J Clin Psychiatry.* 2006;67(5):771-782.

81. Feltner DE, Liu-Dumaw M, Schweizer E, Bielski R. Efficacy of pregabalin in generalized social anxiety disorder: results of a double-blind, placebo-controlled, fixed-dose study. *Int Clin Psychopharmacol.* 2011;26(4):213-220.

82. Greist JH, Liu-Dumaw M, Schweizer E, Feltner D. Efficacy of pregabalin in preventing relapse in patients with generalized social anxiety disorder: results of a double-blind, placebo-controlled 26-week study. *Int Clin Psychopharmacol.* 2011;26(5):243-251.

83. De Salas-Cansado M, Olivares JM, Alvarez E, Carrasco JL, Barrueta A, Rejas J. Pregabalin versus SSRIs and SNRIs in benzodiazepine-refractory outpatients with generalized anxiety disorder: a post hoc cost-effectiveness analysis in usual medical practice in Spain. *Clinicoecon Outcomes Res.* 2012;4:157-168.

84. Urbano MR, Spiegel DR, Laguerta N, Shrader CJ, Rowe DF, Hategan LF. Gabapentin and tiagabine for social anxiety: a randomized, double-blind, crossover study of 8 adults. *Prim Care Companion J Clin Psychiatry.* 2009;11(3):123.

85. Bockbrader HN, Breslin EM, Underwood BA, Posvar EL, Sedman AI. Multiple-dose, dose-proportionality study of neurontin (gabapentin) in healthy volunteers. *Epilepsia.* 1996;37 (suppl 5):159.

86. Cundy KC, Branch R, Chernov-Rogan T. XP13512, a novel gabapentin prodrug: I. Design, synthesis, enzymatic conversion to gabapentin and transport by intestinal solute transporters. *J Pharmacol Exp Ther.* 2004;311(1):315-323.

87. Merlino G, Serafini A, Lorenzut S, Sommaro M, Gigli GL, Valente M. Gabapentin enacarbil in restless legs syndrome. *Drugs Today (Barc).* 2010;46(1):3-11.

88. Kushida CA, Becker PM, Ellenbogen AL, Canafax DM, Barrett RW; XP052 Study Group. Randomized, double-blind, placebo-controlled study of XP13512/GSK1838262 in patients with RLS. *Neurology.* 2009;3;72(5):439-446.

89. Kushida CA, Walters AS, Becker P, et al; XP021 Study Group. A randomized, double-blind, placebo-controlled, crossover study of XP13512/GSK1838262 in the treatment of patients with primary restless legs syndrome. *Sleep.* 2009;1;32(2):159-168.

90. Bogan RK, Bornemann MA, Kushida CA, Trân PV, Barrett RW; XP060 Study Group. Long-term maintenance treatment of restless legs syndrome with gabapentin enacarbil: a randomized controlled study. *Mayo Clin Proc.* 2010;85(6):512-521.

91. Ellenbogen AL, Thein SG, Winslow DH, et al. A 52-week study of gabapentin enacarbil in restless legs syndrome. *Clin Neuropharmacol.* 2011;34(1):8-16.

92. Lee DO, Ziman RB, Perkins AT, Poceta JS, Walters AS, Barrett RW; XP053 Study Group. A randomized, double-blind

placebo-controlled study to assess the efficacy and tolerability of gabapentin enacarbil in subjects with restless legs syndrome. *J Clin Sleep Med.* 2011;7(3):282-292.

93. Winkelman JW, Bogan RK, Schmidt MH, Hudson JD, DeRossett SE, Hill-Zabala CE. Randomized polysomnography study of gabapentin enacarbil in subjects with restless legs syndrome. *Mov Disord.* 2011;26(11):2065-2072.

94. Inoue Y, Uchimura N, Kuroda K, Hirata K, Hattori N. Long-term efficacy and safety of gabapentin enacarbil in Japanese restless legs syndrome patients. *Prog Neuropsychopharmacol Biol Psychiatry.* 2012;36(2):251-257.

95. Mellick GA, Mellick LB. Management of restless legs syndrome with gabapentin (Neurontin) *Sleep.* 1996;19:224-226.

96. Happe S, Klosch G, Saletu B, Zeitlhofer J. Treatment of idiopathic restless legs syndrome (RLS) with gabapentin. *Neurology.* 2001;57:1717-1719.

97. Garcia-Borreguero D, Larrosa O, de la Llave Y, Verger K, Masramon X, Hernandez G. Treatment of restless legs syndrome with gabapentin: a double-blind, cross-over study. *Neurology.* 2002;59:1573-1579.

98. Happe S, Sauter C, Klosch G, Saletu B, Zeitlhofer J. Gabapentin versus ropinirole in the treatment of idiopathic restless legs syndrome. *Neuropsychobiology.* 2003;48:82-86.

99. Saletu M, Anderer P, Saletu-Zyhlarz GM, et al. Comparative placebo-controlled polysomnographic and psychometric studies on the acute effects of gabapentin versus ropinirole in restless legs syndrome. *J Neural Transm.* 2010;117(4):463-473.

100. Thorp ML, Morris CD, Bagby SP. A crossover study of gabapentin in treatment of restless legs syndrome among hemodialysis patients. *Am J Kidney Dis.* 2001;38:104-108.

101. Micozkadioglu H, Ozdemir FN, Kut A, Sezer S, Saatci U, Haberal M. Gabapentin versus levodopa for the treatment of Restless Legs Syndrome in hemodialysis patients: an open-label study. *Ren Fail.* 2004;26:393-397.

102. Sommer M, Bachmann CG, Liebetanz KM, Schindehutte J, Tings T, Paulus W. Pregabalin in restless legs syndrome with and without neuropathic pain. *Acta Neurol Scand.* 2007;115: 347-350.

103. Garcia-Borreguero D, Larrosa O, Williams AM, et al. Treatment of restless legs syndrome with pregabalin: a double-blind, placebo-controlled study. *Neurology.* 2010;74(23):1897-1904.

104. Allen R, Chen C, Soaita A. A randomized, double-blind, 6-week, dose-ranging study of pregabalin in patients with restless legs syndrome. *Sleep Med*. 2010;11(6):512-519.

105. Telstad W, Sørensen O, Larsen S, Lillevold PE, Stensrud P, Nyberg-Hansen R. Treatment of the restless legs syndrome with carbamazepine: a double blind study. *Br Med J (Clin Res Ed)*. 1984;288(6415):444-446.

106. Sørensen O, Telstad W. Carbamazepine (Tegretol) in restless legs [in Norwegian]. *Tidsskr Nor Laegeforen*. 1984;104:2093-2095.

107. Larsen S, Telstad W, Sørensen O, Thom E, Stensrud P, Nyberg-Hansen R. Carbamazepine therapy in restless legs. Discrimination between responders and non-responders. *Acta Med Scand*. 1985;218:223-227.

108. Youssef EA, Wagner ML, Martinez JO, Hening W. Pilot trial of lamotrigine in the restless legs syndrome. *Sleep Med*. 2005;6:89.

109. Della Marca G, Vollono C, Mariotti P, et al. Levetiracetam can be effective in the treatment of restless legs syndrome with periodic limb movements in sleep: report of two cases. *J Neurol Neurosurg Psychiatry*. 2006;77:566-567.

110. Ozturk O, Eraslan D, Kumral E. Oxcarbazepine treatment for paroxetine-induced restless leg syndrome. *Gen Hosp Psychiatry*. 2006;28:264-265.

111. Perez Bravo A. Topiramate use as treatment in restless legs syndrome. *Actas Esp Psiquiatr*. 2004;32:132-137.

112. Eisensehr I, Ehrenberg BL, Rogge Solti S, Noachtar S. Treatment of idiopathic restless legs syndrome (RLS) with slow-release valproic acid compared with slow-release levodopa/benserazid. *J Neurol*. 2004;251:579-583.

113. Ekbom KA. Restless legs syndrome. *Neurology*. 1960;10:868-873.

114. Trzepacz PT, Violette EJ, Sateia MJ. Response to opioids in three patients with restless legs syndrome. *Am J Psychiatry*. 1984;141:993-995.

115. Walters A, Hening W, Cote L, Fahn S. Dominantly inherited restless legs with myoclonus and periodic movements of sleep: a syndrome related to the endogenous opiates? *Adv Neurol*. 1986;43:309-19.

116. Sandyk R, Gillman MA. The opioid system in the restless legs and nocturnal myoclonus syndromes. *Sleep*. 1986;9:370-371.

9

117. Hening WA, Walters A, Kavey N, Gidro-Frank S, Cote L, Fahn S. Dyskinesias while awake and periodic movements in sleep in restless legs syndrome: treatment with opioids. *Neurology.* 1986;36:1363-1366.

118. Winkelmann J, Schadrack J, Wetter TC, Zieglgansberger W, Trenkwalder C. Opioid and dopamine antagonist drug challenges in untreated restless legs syndrome patients. *Sleep Med.* 2001;2:57-61.

119. Walters AS. Review of receptor agonist and antagonist studies relevant to the opiate system in restless legs syndrome. *Sleep Med.* 2002;3:301-304.

120. Montplaisir J, Lorrain D, Godbout R. Restless legs syndrome and periodic leg movements in sleep: the primary role of dopaminergic mechanism. *Eur Neurol.* 1991;31:41-43.

121. Aurora RN, Kristo DA, Bista SR, et al. The treatment of restless legs syndrome and periodic limb movement disorder in adults-an update for 2012: practice parameters with an evidence-based systematic review and meta-analysis: an American Academy of Sleep Medicine Clinical Practice Guideline. *Sleep.* 2012;35(8):1039-1062.

122. Walters AS, Winkelmann J, Trenkwalder C, et al. Long-term follow-up on restless legs syndrome patients treated with opioids. *Mov Disord.* 2001;16:1105-1109.

123. Dayer P, Collart L, Desmeules J. The pharmacology of tramadol. *Drugs.* 1994;47(suppl 1):3-7.

124. Preston KL, Jasinski DR, Testa M. Abuse potential and pharmacological comparison of tramadol and morphine. *Drug Alcohol Depend.* 1991;27:7-17.

125. Cicero TJ, Inciardi JA, Adams EH, et al. Rates of abuse of tramadol remain unchanged with the introduction of new branded and generic products: results of an abuse monitoring system, 1994-2004. *Pharmacoepidemiol Drug Saf.* 2005;14:851-859.

126. Adams EH, Breiner S, Cicero TJ, et al. A comparison of the abuse liability of tramadol, NSAIDs, and hydrocodone in patients with chronic pain. *J Pain Symptom Manage.* 2006;31:465-476.

127. Lauerma H, Markkula J. Treatment of restless legs syndrome with tramadol: an open study. *J Clin Psychiatry.* 1999;60:241-244.

128. Ondo WG. Methadone for refractory restless legs syndrome. *Mov Disord.* 2005;20:345-348.

129. Silver N, Allen RP, Senerth J, Earley CJ. A 10-year, longitudinal assessment of dopamine agonists and methadone in the treatment of restless legs syndrome. *Sleep Med*. 2011; 12(5):440-444.

130. Davis MP, Walsh D. Methadone for relief of cancer pain: a review of pharmacokinetics, pharmacodynamics, drug interactions and protocols of administration. *Support Care Cancer*. 2001;9:73-83.

131. Sees KL, Delucchi KL, Masson C, et al. Methadone maintenance vs 180-day psychosocially enriched detoxification for treatment of opioid dependence: a randomized controlled trial. *JAMA*. 2000;283:1303-1310.

132. Blake AD, Bot G, Freeman JC, Reisine T. Differential opioid agonist regulation of the mouse mu opioid receptor. *J Biol Chem*. 1997;272:782-790.

133. Jakobsson B, Ruuth K. Successful treatment of restless legs syndrome with an implanted pump for intrathecal drug delivery. *Acta Anaesthesiol Scand*. 2002;46:114-117.

134. Vahedi H, Küchle M, Trenkwalder C, Krenz CJ. Peridural morphine administration in restless legs status [in German] [published correction appears in *Anasthesiol Intensivmed Notfallmed Schmerzther* 1994;29(8):521]. *Anasthesiol Intensivmed Notfallmed Schmerzther*. 1994;29(6):368-370.

135. Walters AS, Wagner ML, Hening WA, et al. Successful treatment of the idiopathic restless legs syndrome in a randomized double-blind trial of oxycodone versus placebo. *Sleep*. 1993;16:327-332.

136. Matthews WB. Treatment of the restless legs syndrome with clonazepam. *Br Med J*. 1979;1:751.

137. Allen RP, Picchietti D, Hening WA, Trenkwalder C, Walters AS, Montplaisi J; Restless Legs Syndrome Diagnosis and Epidemiology workshop at the National Institutes of Health; International Restless Legs Syndrome Study Group. Restless legs syndrome: diagnostic criteria, special considerations, and epidemiology. A report from the restless legs syndrome diagnosis and epidemiology workshop at the National Institutes of Health. *Sleep Med*. 2003;4:101-119.

138. Allen RP, Lesage S, Earley CJ. Anti-histamines and benzodiazepines exacerbate daytime restless legs syndrome (RLS) symptoms. *Sleep*. 2005;28:A279. Abstract.

139. Mitler MM, Browman CP, Menn SJ, Gujavarty K, Timms RM. Nocturnal myoclonus: treatment efficacy of clonazepam and temazepam. *Sleep*. 1986;9:385-392.

9

140. Scharf MB, Brown L, Hirschowitz J. Possible efficacy of alprazolam in restless leg syndrome. *Hillside J Clin Psychiatry*. 1986;8:214-223.

141. Boghen D. Successful treatment of restless legs with clonazepam. *Ann Neurol*. 1980;8:341.

142. Montagna P, Sassoli de Bianchi L, Zucconi M, Cirignotta F, Lugaresi E. Clonazepam and vibration in restless legs syndrome. *Acta Neurol Scand*. 1984;69:428-430.

143. Boghen D, Lamothe L, Elie R, Godbout R, Montplaisir J. The treatment of the restless legs syndrome with clonazepam: a prospective controlled study. *Can J Neurol Sci*. 1986;13:245-247.

144. Tollefson G, Erdman C. Triazolam in the restless legs syndrome. *J Clin Psychopharmacol*. 1985;5:361-362.

145. Doghramji K, Browman CP, Gaddy JR, Walsh JK. Triazolam diminishes daytime sleepiness and sleep fragmentation in patients with periodic leg movements in sleep. *J Clin Psychopharmacol*. 1991;11:284-290.

146. Bonnet MH, Arand DL. Chronic use of triazolam in patients with periodic leg movements, fragmented sleep and daytime sleepiness. *Aging (Milano)*. 1991;3(4):313-324.

147. Borja NL, Daniel KL. Ramelteon for the treatment of insomnia. *Clin Ther*. 2006;28:1540-1555.

148. Bezerra ML, Martinez JV. Zolpidem in restless legs syndrome. *Eur Neurol*. 2002;48:180-181.

149. Morgenthaler TI, Silber MH. Amnestic sleep-related eating disorder associated with zolpidem. *Sleep Med*. 2002;3:323-327.

150. Evidente VG, Adler CH, Caviness JN, Hentz JG, Gwinn-Hardy K. Amantadine is beneficial in restless legs syndrome. *Mov Disord*. 2000;15:324-327.

151. Rotenberg JS, Canard K, Difazio M. Successful treatment of recalcitrant restless legs syndrome with botulinum toxin type-A. *J Clin Sleep Med*. 2006;2:275-278.

152. Handwerker JV Jr, Palmer RF. Clonidine in the treatment of "restless leg" syndrome. *N Engl J Med*. 1985;313:1228-1229.

153. Cavatorta F, Vagge R, Solari P, Queirolo C. Preliminary results with clonidine in the restless legs syndrome in 2 hemodialyzed uremic patients. *Minerva Urol Nefrol*. 1987;39:93.

154. Bastani B, Westervelt FB. Effectiveness of clonidine in alleviating the symptoms of "restless legs". *Am J Kidney Dis*. 1987;10:326.

155. Zoe A, Wagner ML, Walters AS. High-dose clonidine in a case of restless legs syndrome. *Ann Pharmacother*. 1994;28:878-881.

156. Wagner ML, Walters AS, Coleman RG, Hening WA, Grasing K, Chokroverty S. Randomized, double-blind, placebo-controlled study of clonidine in restless legs syndrome. *Sleep*. 1996;19:52-58.

157. Bamford CR, Sandyk R. Failure of clonidine to ameliorate the symptoms of restless legs syndrome. *Sleep*. 1987;10:398-399.

158. Strang RR. The symptom of restless legs. *Med J Aust*. 1967;1: 1211-1213.

159. Lipinski JF, Zubenko GS, Barreira P, Cohen BM. Propranolol in the treatment of neuroleptic-induced akathisia. *Lancet*. 1983;2:685-686.

160. Derom E, Elinck W, Buylaert W, van der Straeten M. Which beta-blocker for the restless leg? *Lancet*. 1984;1:857.

161. Ginsberg HN. Propranolol in the treatment of restless legs syndrome induced by imipramine withdrawal. *Am J Psychiatry*. 1986;143:938.

162. O'Sullivan RL, Greenberg DB. H2 antagonists, restless leg syndrome, and movement disorders. *Psychosomatics*. 1993; 34:530-532.

163. Botez MI. Folate deficiency and neurological disorders in adults. *Med Hypotheses*. 1976;2:135-140.

164. Botez MI, Cadotte M, Beaulieu R, Pichette LP, Pison C. Neurologic disorders responsive to folic acid therapy. *Can Med Assoc J*. 1976;115:217-223.

165. Ayres S Jr, Mihan R. Leg cramps (systremma) and "restless legs" syndrome. Response to vitamin E (tocopherol). *Calif Med*. 1969;111:87-91.

166. Ayres S Jr, Mihan R. Restless legs syndrome: response to vitamin E. *J Appl Nutr* 1973;25:8-15.

167. Botez MI, Fontaine F, Botez T, Bachevalier J. Folate-responsive neurological and mental disorders: report of 16 cases. Neuropsychological correlates of computerized transaxial tomography and radionuclide cisternography in folic acid deficiencies. *Eur Neurol*. 1977;16:230-246.

168. Lee KA, Zaffke ME, Baratte-Beebe K. Restless legs syndrome and sleep disturbance during pregnancy: the role of folate and iron. *J Womens Health Gend Based Med*. 2001;10:335-341.

169. Bateman PP. The "restless legs" syndrome. *Med J Aust*. 1991; 155:135.

9

170. Hornyak M, Voderholzer U, Hohagen F, Berger M, Riemann D. Magnesium therapy for periodic leg movements-related insomnia and restless legs syndrome: an open pilot study. *Sleep*. 1998;21:501-505.

171. Walters AS, Elin RJ, Cohen B, Moller JC, Oertel W, Stiasny-Kolster K. Magnesium not likely to play a major role in the pathogenesis of Restless Legs Syndrome: serum and cerebrospinal fluid studies. *Sleep Med*. 2007;8:186-187.

10 Approaching the Patient with RLS

Although people with restless legs syndrome (RLS) may seem symptomatically quite similar at first, they are actually a diverse group of patients who often present with different needs for treatment. To help decide on the most appropriate of the available therapies, several algorithms have been constructed to help guide physicians to a practical approach to treating RLS patients.[1-8]

A number of these algorithms categorize the treatment based on the frequency of symptoms, which tends to be an effective starting point. Suggestions from most of these articles are considered in this chapter, but the treatment recommendation is patterned most closely on the algorithms discussed in the more recent articles. These algorithms are further augmented with practical suggestions based on considerable clinical experience.

Patients with Intermittent Symptoms

Intermittent RLS is defined as symptoms when not treated would occur on average <2/week for the past year with at least 5 lifetime events. People with intermittent symptoms represent the largest group of those with RLS. They embody a wide spectrum of the disease with symptoms that may occur once every few months to less than twice weekly. As such, they often need somewhat different therapy based on the frequency, time of day, and intensity of symptoms.

In general, people with intermittent RLS tend to have milder symptoms and respond more readily to treatment than those with daily symptoms. Therefore, this group of patients is usually easier to treat. However, as they are still quite a diverse group, treatment should be individualized as discussed below.

The general approach to treating these patients is detailed in the algorithm for the management of intermittent RLS in **Figure 10.1**. Often, the RLS symptoms may respond to nonpharmacologic therapies (see *Chapter 8*) and totally avoid the need for drugs. However, even if these non-drug therapies are successful, there may still be occasions when these techniques are not adequate and medication may be necessary. It is often wise to prescribe as-needed (prn) medication for sporadic use when the non-drug therapies are not sufficient. The selection for an as needed medication is detailed in **Table 10.1**.

FIGURE 10.1 — Algorithm for the Management of Intermittent RLS

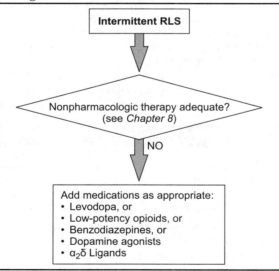

- **Instituting Nonpharmacologic Therapy**

Avoid Medications That Worsen RLS

Physicians should start by reviewing the patient's medication list, including medications that are taken on an as-needed basis and over-the-counter ones. When

TABLE 10.1 — Drugs for Intermittent RLS

Type of RLS Problem	Suitable Drugs
Bedtime RLS	
Infrequent	Sedative/hypnotics, opioid analgesics, or L-dopa
≥3 nights/week	Approved dopamine agonists or α2δ ligands
Daytime RLS	
Expected	Dopamine agonists, L-dopa, α2δ ligands ,opioid analgesics
Unexpected	Opioid analgesics or L-dopa
One drug fits all needs	Opioid analgesics or L-dopa

possible, drugs that worsen RLS should be changed to more RLS-friendly ones (see *Chapter 8* and *Chapter 12*). Patients should be advised to obtain an RLS medical-alert card (available from the RLS Foundation) so that they can be aware of these medications and also inform their physicians who may not be as knowledgeable about the disorder.

10

Abstinence from Alcohol, Caffeine, and Nicotine

There should be a review of dietary and other habits to help eliminate alcohol, caffeine, and nicotine. Counseling and other treatments may be necessary to help patients avoid these often addictive behaviors.

Develop a "Bag of Tricks"

Patients should be advised to plan for situations that worsen RLS. For example, stimulating activities may be helpful for sedentary situations (eg, airplane trips) that typically trigger RLS. They may need to bring a deck of cards, hand-held video game, crossword puzzle, or other mentally engaging activities when going on trips. However, many other activities (eg, stretches, exercise, hot or cold baths, and other counterstimulation activities) may alleviate RLS symptoms. Patients should be advised to develop a large bag of tricks that contains a variety of techniques to help cope with all of the diverse situations that may trigger or worsen RLS.

Sleep Hygiene

Proper sleep hygiene is often essential for RLS patients to minimize their symptoms. As with insomnia, which occurs frequently in RLS patients, it is important to review the rules of sleep hygiene (discussed in *Chapter 8*) and ensure that patients are getting adequate sleep.

Exercise

Mild-to-moderate levels of exercise have been demonstrated to improve RLS symptoms.[9] Patients should be counseled to perform regular (at least three to four times per week) exercise that may help their RLS and provide other health benefits.

Education and Support Groups

RLS patients should be encouraged to join the RLS Foundation (www.rls.org) and, if available, a local support group. This involvement teaches patients about RLS and they can learn how to live with their disease. Speaking with other RLS patients often gives them insights on how to deal with friends, family, and coworkers and may be an invaluable resource for adding to their bag of tricks. In addition, there are many Web sites with information on RLS as well as forums and chat groups that can benefit RLS patients (see *Appendix B*).

Iron Therapy

RLS patients should have their serum ferritin level checked even when their hemoglobin and serum iron levels are normal. The serum ferritin level is the most accurate and sensitive test (other than a bone marrow evaluation) to determine whether iron stores are low. Serum ferritin levels <50-75 ug/mL (despite lab-reported normal levels of >10-20 ug/mL) have been associated with an increased severity of RLS,[10,11] and treating these patients with supplemental iron may help their RLS. For further discussion on the administration of iron therapy for RLS, see Secondary RLS in *Chapter 11*.

■ Instituting Drug Therapy for Intermittent RLS

Even patients with mild, infrequent RLS symptoms have occasions when the non-drug therapies discussed are not sufficient and medication may be needed. Their RLS may be exacerbated by a long airplane trip, medication, anxiety, or many other triggers. As noted, it is helpful to prescribe as-needed medication for most RLS patients.

As of now, no medications are approved for as-needed use for the treatment of intermittent RLS and studies of intermittent RLS are rare. However, expert opinions based on significant clinical experience can provide some suggestions for managing these patients. Medications for those with intermittent RLS can be chosen from the algorithm in **Figure 10**.1 and guided by **Table 10**.1. The choice of medication should match the frequency and timing of the symptoms. For example, it is clear that a sedative hypnotic drug may be appropriate for bedtime RLS but not for daytime symptoms.

Infrequent Bedtime RLS (<2 nights/week)

Bedtime presents significant problems for most RLS sufferers. Symptoms tend to peak and effective treatment should be initiated promptly to avoid increased anxiety that may further hamper sleep onset. Therefore, a quick-acting agent is the most appropriate choice in this situation.

Which of the drugs listed in **Table 10**.1 for infrequent bedtime RLS is the best choice for this situation? They are all reasonable choices and it depends more upon how well the drug works for the individual patient and the comfort level of the physician prescribing them.

Any of the sedative hypnotic drugs are suitable for bedtime RLS symptoms; most of them have a rapid onset and typically accomplish the main goal of enabling the patient to fall asleep. As per the discussion of these drugs in *Chapter 9,* hypnotics with a shorter half-life are a better choice, although if sleep maintenance is a concern, drugs with a somewhat longer half-life may be warranted. There is also less concern about tolerance and dependence when using these drugs on an intermittent basis.

Opioid analgesics, which include the opioids and tramadol (see *Chapter 9*) are also effective for treating bedtime RLS. They tend to onset quickly and are usually quite potent for relieving RLS symptoms. As with the sedative hypnotics, there is less concern about tolerance and dependence when using them intermittently. Typically, the low to medium potency opioids (codeine, one half to 1 tablet of hydrocodone or tramadol) are appropriate in this setting.

L-dopa containing drugs (carbidopa/L-dopa or benserazide/L-dopa) are also good choices in this situation. These drugs have a quick onset, typically within 30 minutes or as fast as 15 minutes on an empty stomach. There is no concern about augmentation with L-dopa when used on an intermittent basis.

Frequent Bedtime RLS (≥2 nights/week)

Although this falls under the category of chronic-persistent RLS, treatment options similar to intermittent RLS may be more appropriate for some patients depending upon the frequency and intensity of symptoms. For patients with more frequent (even with daily occurring) RLS symptoms that are mild enough not to disturb sleep on a routine basis, drug choices should be similar to the choices above for infrequent bedtime RLS. These patients can go to bed then wait to see if their RLS symptoms prevent going to sleep. When that happens, any of the medications mentioned in the section above should be helpful to get them to sleep quickly.

However, when more intense, bothersome RLS symptoms occur twice weekly or more, daily treatment should be considered. Not treating disruptive, severe RLS symptoms may create significant anxiety and initiate a chronic insomnia problem. Thus, it may be appropriate to treat these patients preemptively with daily medication, as per **Table 10**.**1**, which may help abort the anxiety/insomnia cycle. Clearly, this is a more complex decision that should be discussed at length with the patient with the purpose of fashioning a plan of treatment tailored to their individual needs.

Expected Daytime RLS

Many people with intermittent RLS can easily predict when their RLS will typically worsen and require drug treatment for such situations. Common examples are evening movies or airplane trips. Patients can plan to take medication before symptoms occur. This is generally a good idea as it avoids any suffering and lower doses are often effective when taken prior to the onset of symptoms.

The dopamine agonists are a reasonable choice for this situation as they can be taken 1 to 3 hours prior to the provocation and, due to their long half-life, can protect patients for prolonged situations, such as airplane or other trips. The $\alpha_2\delta$ ligands may also be helpful but sedation (especially when used on an intermittent basis) may be an issue for activities such as going to the movies or theater. However, they might be helpful for a long airplane flight if the patient would rather sleep through it.

Some patients may prefer to wait and see if symptoms occur or can be eliminated with non-drug therapy. For those patients, the quicker-acting opioid analgesics (low-potency opioids or tramadol) and L-dopa may be reasonable. These drugs can also be used prophylactically before situations of shorter duration that exacerbate RLS. Analgesic drugs may cause daytime sedation and, therefore, may be inappropriate for some individuals and for activities that require alertness, such as theater or other public entertainment.

The best drug for this situation is the one that the patient tolerates, is effective, and fits their needs. In some cases, it may take some trial and error to determine the proper choice of therapy.

Unexpected Daytime RLS

Despite the best planning and intentions, there will be situations that occur when patients forget to take their medications prophylactically or symptoms just appear at unexpected times. This situation is similar to infrequent bedtime RLS in that quick relief is necessary. Therefore, the choice of drug is also similar, except that the sedative hypnotic drugs are usually inappropriate, as alertness is impaired. An exception may be a long airplane flight. However, if the person is awakened in flight (eg, when served a meal), RLS symptoms may promptly return.

Therefore, the choice is usually between the opioid analgesics (low-potency opioids or tramadol) and L-dopa. Again, the correct drug is the one that is best tolerated, most effective, and fits the patient's needs.

One Drug Fits All Needs

Many patients may fit into one of the described categories, but commonly patients have multiple needs. RLS symptoms may appear unpredictably at odd times and cause both daytime and bedtime problems. Physicians may also need to treat more predictable exacerbating factors (eg, addressing medications which provoke RLS).

Although some patients may prefer to have an arsenal of medications to treat their RLS in all of the different potential situations, it may be simpler to prescribe one medication that can be used in all the described situations. Opioid analgesics and L-dopa fit most of these needs fairly well. Either of these drugs is a good choice for patients who have intermittent RLS that does not warrant regular medication. These medications are also good choices for as-needed use in patients who need daily medication and in those who rely on non-drug therapy but may need medication on rare occasions. The latter group of patients may be thankful to have drugs available for those unusual times when nothing else works.

Chronic-persistent/daily RLS is defined by untreated symptoms occurring on average at least twice a week for the past year. Most of the patients in this category will have more severe symptoms than those with intermittent RLS and symptoms may be difficult to control with non-drug therapy. However, as per the algorithm in **Figure 10.2**, nonpharmacologic therapy (see *Chapter 9*) should be the first approach and many of the patients with less intense and infrequent symptoms may respond adequately to these measures. When this treatment is unsuccessful at effectively relieving RLS symptoms, drug therapy should be considered.

Patients with symptoms that occur less than daily or whose symptoms occur daily but are not always disruptive may be treated somewhat similar to those with intermittent RLS symptoms. It is likely that the majority of the patients in this category will not be satisfied with this treatment but it may work for a significant percentage of them and is worth considering. However, for patients with more persistent intense and bothersome symptoms, especially when they occur almost daily, drug therapy is usually necessary.

■ Choice of Initial Drug Therapy

Prior to 2011 when gabapentin enacarbil was approved, the choice of first-line treatment was more straightforward, including only the two short-acting dopamine agonists, pramipexole and ropinirole. Now that there are more approved drugs, that decision has become more complex. **Table 10.2** is an excellent guide prepared by a task force from the IRLSSG (International RLS Study Group)[12] that should help guide a physician to the best drug based upon the characteristics of the drugs and the needs and comorbidities of the patient. Most of those recommendations are discussed below.

FIGURE 10.2 — Algorithm for the Management of Chronic-Persistent/Daily RLS

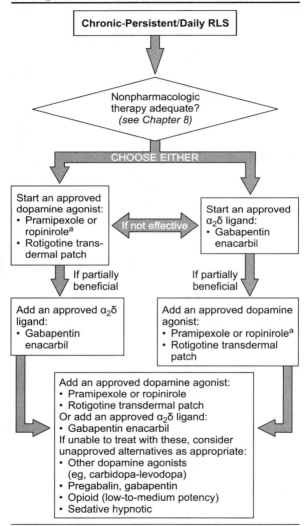

ᵃ Patients should be educated about the risk of developing augmentation with these short-acting dopamine agonists.

TABLE 10.2 — Factors That Affect Selection of an Agent for Initial Treatment in Patients With RLS/WED

Factor That Impacts the Choice of Agent	Treatment Choice
Time of day (daytime disturbance)	Preferably a long-acting agent; twice-a-day dosing of a short-acting agent
Sleep disturbance disproportionate to other symptoms of RLS/WED, eg, very severe and symptomatic insomnia	$\alpha 2\delta$ Ligand
Comorbid insomnia	$\alpha 2\delta$ Ligand
Pregnancy risk	Avoid both DAs and $\alpha 2\delta$ ligands; consider the use of iron
Impaired renal function	Select a drug that is not renally excreted
Increased risk of falls	Dopamine-receptor agonist
Painful restless legs	$\alpha 2\delta$ Ligand
Comorbid pain syndrome	$\alpha 2\delta$ Ligand
History of ICD	$\alpha 2\delta$ Ligand
History of alcohol or substance abuse	Dopamine-receptor agonist or $\alpha 2\delta$ ligand
Very severe symptoms of RLS/WED	Dopamine-receptor agonist
Excess weight, metabolic syndrome, or obstructive sleep apnea	Dopamine-receptor agonist
Comorbid depression	Dopamine-receptor agonist
Comorbid generalized anxiety disorder	$\alpha 2\delta$ Ligand
Daytime sleepiness	Investigate the cause
Higher potential for drug interactions	Select drug that is not hepatically excreted

10

Summary of Recommendations for the Long-Term Treatment of RLS/WED from an IRLSSG Task Force. International Restless Legs Syndrome Study Group Web site. http://irlssg.org/summary. Accessed March 13, 2013.

Although the two approved short-acting dopamine agonists act somewhat differently on the dopamine subtype receptors, they are reasonably similar in their efficacy and side effect profile when treating RLS. Ropinirole may have a little faster onset than pramipexole but its duration of action is shorter (half-life of 6 hours compared with 8 to 12 hours for pramipexole). Ropinirole is approximately one half to one fourth as potent as pramipexole on an mg basis but this is also reflected in the strength of pills available for each drug. Ropinirole is metabolized by the liver while pramipexole is excreted through the kidneys so patients with organ damage may do better with the drug that does not depend on that organ for elimination.

For most patients, both drugs may be appropriate and the choice should be based upon the physician's experience and comfort level with these drugs. Both of these drugs are available in less expensive generic forms which is helpful when financial concerns are present. However, many RLS experts are now advocating that these drugs not be dosed at their FDA-approved upper limit, but rather at much lower levels (1 mg for ropinirole, 0.25 mg for pramipexole).

The concern with short-acting dopamine agonists is that augmentation may be more common than previously thought. This is a significant issue since RLS is a lifelong disease and these drugs will be used for decades, increasing the odds of augmentation occurring eventually. Therefore, when considering the use of a dopamine agonist, it may be prudent to choose a long-acting one (eg, rotigotine transdermal patch). This drug may be more appropriate for long-term therapy due to its long duration of action likely resulting in less augmentation issues. Furthermore, although many RLS patients do not complain about their daytime symptoms, they are often impaired by them and simply adjust their lifestyle to work through these symptoms.

A recent study[13] found that 69% of patients with moderate to severe RLS had breakthrough daytime RLS which often occurred unexpectedly. Thus, providing a drug that covers symptoms around the clock should be beneficial for many RLS patients with chronic-persistent symptoms and gives them more freedom from worrying about daytime RLS symptoms occurring during sedentary activities. Of course, for patients who present with daytime symptoms in addition to the usual evening/nighttime ones, rotigotine is an excellent and preferred selection.

Since the approval of gabapentin enacarbil in 2011, the choice of first-line treatment has been divided between the dopamine agonists and this $\alpha2\delta$ ligand. Numerous studies have proven gabapentin enacarbil to be effective and safe for treating moderate to severe RLS (see *Chapter 9*). The advantage of this drug is that it does not cause augmentation and also may help insomnia, which is very common in RLS patients. However, the sedative effect which typically peaks at bedtime may cause evening sleepiness or next day sleepiness that can impair their awake-time activities for some patients.

In patients with painful RLS symptoms or with comorbid chronic pain syndrome, such as postherpetic neuralgia, gabapentin enacarbil would also be a preferred option. Patients with a history of an impulse control disorder should not be given dopamine agonist drugs and would be better suited for an $\alpha2\delta$ ligand. However, since anticonvulsant drugs may cause suicidal ideation, patients with severe depression should be started on these medications with caution.

■ Choice of Secondary Drug Therapy

If the patient cannot take the above approved first-line drugs due to intolerance, lack of efficacy, cost, or availability, then the second-line medications may be considered. Replacing approved dopamine agonists is more difficult as most of the remaining ones are ergot-derived and the risk of fibrotic heart valve damage outweighs the benefits (except perhaps when no other options are available). However, the two long-acting dopamine agonists, pramipexole ER and ropinirole XL, may be appropriate for patients who had problems with the shorter-acting ones. However, they have not yet been studied for treating RLS and are not FDA approved for the treatment of RLS. Theoretically, they may cover RLS symptoms for longer periods and more steady blood levels that may result in fewer side effects. Also, coverage may be limited as these medications are only approved for treating Parkinson's disease.

When patients cannot take gabapentin enacarbil, alternatives include gabapentin and pregabalin. These drugs act upon the same receptors as gabapentin enacarbil and tend to have similar side effect profiles. Gabapentin has the advantage of being inexpensive, readily available, and physicians have experience using it. However, it is not equivalent to using gabapentin enacarbil as discussed in *Chapter 9* and typically results in unpredictable doses and treatment effects. If no other $\alpha2\delta$ ligands are affordable or available, this drug may be considered. Pregabalin's relatively short action (half-life of 6 hours) may be beneficial for some patients who have shorter episodes of RLS symptoms or wish to use differential split doses with lower doses earlier in the day to decrease their total daily dose. Patients who need two to three doses per day may find longer-acting drugs more convenient. Pregabalin is approved for the treatment of generalized anxiety disorder by the European Commission. Therefore, it may be a viable option for RLS patients with anxiety issues.

There are few studies on the non-$\alpha2\delta$ ligand anticonvulsants but they may be helpful in sporadic cases that do not respond to the $\alpha2\delta$ ligands or when the $\alpha2\delta$ ligands are not available or affordable. Clinical experience has found that although most patients do not respond as well to the non-$\alpha2\delta$ ligand anticonvulsants, sporadic cases may benefit from their use.

Typically, the use of opioids and sedative hypnotics for patients with chronic-persistent RLS are best as add-on supplemental therapies for first-line drugs.

Opioids are helpful for daytime symptoms (especially when combined with drugs that are taken later in the day for the more common evening/nighttime symptoms) or for breakthrough or unexpected symptoms that need quick relief. Typically, these drugs are used more on an intermittent basis but may also be prescribed on a daily basis for patients who have not achieved full relief with the use of first-line drugs. Combination therapy (see below) is often helpful to keep the doses of drugs at lower levels that may make them more tolerable and decrease the chances of long-term problems such as augmentation. The low to medium potency opioids are most suited for treating this class of patients. Opioids should be avoided in patients with a history of drug abuse and used with caution in patients with sleep apnea (especially central sleep apnea) and chronic obstructive pulmonary disease due to the potential for respiratory depression.

Even when RLS symptoms are completely resolved with first-line drugs, patients should be questioned about how well they are sleeping as chronic insomnia often persists. Many of these patients may benefit from a sedative hypnotic sleeping pill. Intermittent use of sleeping pills is safer as it prevents the emergence of tolerance and dependence. If patients need them on a daily basis, proper sleep hygiene and cognitive-behavioral therapy should be instituted to help reduce their daily use. As discussed in *Chapter 9*, the shorter-acting sedatives and non-benzodiazepines are typically preferred.

Patients With Refractory RLS

Refractory RLS is defined as chronic-persistent/daily RLS that has failed available first-line therapy (at least one adequate trial of a first-line, approved dopamine agonist and also an α2δ ligand) with one or more of the following outcomes:

- Inadequate initial response despite adequate doses
- Response that has become inadequate with time, despite increasing doses
- Intolerable adverse effects
- Augmentation that is not controllable with additional earlier doses of the drug.

These patients include the most difficult to manage RLS patients. Since few studies have been performed to determine how these patients should be treated, the recommendations in this section are based on the considerable experience of experts in the field. Once all the approved drugs have been tried and failed, the physician is left with considering the use of non-approved drugs. **Figure 10.3** provides a general schema that illustrates some of the useful therapeutic strategies that have worked for those experienced with managing these patients. As primary care physicians become more familiar with RLS, they should be able to care for many of these patients, especially with the aid of this section. However, referral to an RLS specialist may be an appropriate option when patients are not responding to treatment as expected or when physicians are not comfortable and/or knowledgeable enough to use all the available medications.

Each of the situations resulting in refractory RLS will be discussed and specific suggestions provided for them. Following the suggestions should aid physicians to treat a significant number of these more difficult RLS patients.

■ Inadequate Initial Response Despite Adequate Doses of Approved Dopamine Agonists and/or α2δ Ligand

As discussed, dopamine agonists should be started at the lowest available dose then increased slowly until symptoms are relieved. Since >90% of RLS patients respond to dopaminergic drugs,[14] only a small percentage will fall into the category of refractory RLS. Although some patients seem to respond only to high

FIGURE 10.3 — Algorithm for the Management of Refractory RLS

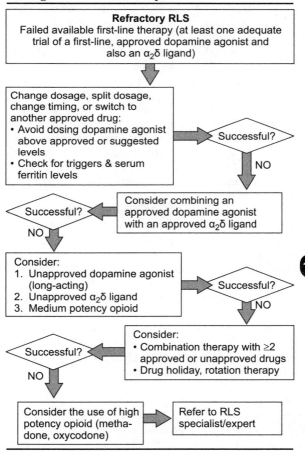

doses of these drugs, most do well with the lower/ average dose ranges tabulated in **Table 9.3**. Physicians should be careful in exceeding the typical dose ranges of dopaminergics, as further titration will probably eventually result in more side effects than relief.

Once reasonable doses of the drug have proved ineffective, other strategies need to be considered.

247

Often, if one dopamine agonist lacks efficacy, another one may work better. Patients clearly differ in their responses to these drugs, so if one does not help, another should be tried before giving up on this class.

If dopamine agonists provide no relief, then approved α2δ ligands (currently only gabapentin enacarbil) should be tried as detailed in *Chapter 9*. Of course, the reverse is true if α2δ ligands are tried first and fail, then dopamine agonists should be prescribed.

If the dopamine agonist or α2δ ligand each helps somewhat but does not completely relieve all of the RLS symptoms, treating with the combination of these two classes of medication can be beneficial. Furthermore, adding a sedative hypnotic may be helpful for insomnia from bedtime RLS that does not fully respond to dopamine drugs and/or α2δ ligands.

If there is inadequate relief provided from approved dopamine agonists and α2δ ligands (alone and/or in combination), the use of unapproved dopamine agonist and α2δ ligands or medium potency opioids may be considered next. The majority of patients typically respond to opioids and often they can be used successfully as monotherapy. If there have been partial responses to approved dopamine agonists and/or α2δ ligands, they can be added for cases in which patients are not fully responding to opioid monotherapy. The alternative selection (before trying opioids) of unapproved dopamine agonists and α2δ ligands may be considered and may provide relief when the approved ones have failed (although this is less common). These drugs can also be combined with medium potency opioids for patients requiring combination therapy.

As per **Figure 10**.**3**, if the above therapy does not work, then high potency opioids should be strongly considered. Most patients, even those who have not responded adequately to medium potency opioids will usually benefit from the high potency opioids. Many RLS experts prefer to start with methadone when a high potency opioid is needed as it seems to be more effective and tolerated in this setting. As discussed in *Chapter 9*, with proper patient selection, monitoring, and dosing, tolerance/dependence and addiction should not occur. Furthermore, as also discussed in *Chapter 9*, the American Academy of Sleep Medicine recommended that opioids should be considered as a guideline treatment for RLS in their 2012 article for practice guidelines for the management of RLS.[15] When these drugs are necessary to treat refractory RLS, they should not be withheld from patients due to the above concerns. Physicians not able or willing to prescribe long-term opioids should refer these patients to specialists who can take care of them properly.

■ Response That Has Become Inadequate With Time Despite Increasing Doses

Many patients initially respond well to dopamine agonists and α2δ ligands. However, over time (typically many months to years), this response may wane. Whether this is due to the worsening of RLS by a new trigger, tolerance to the drug, or the natural progression of the disease is often difficult to discern. Regardless of the etiology, this can be a difficult problem to solve.

Worsening Due to a New Trigger

It is not uncommon for RLS patients to be prescribed medications that worsen RLS, such as antidepressants. Therefore, when patients present with a diminished response to therapy, it is always worthwhile to review their complete medication list (both prescription and over the counter) thoroughly. Often prescription changes can be made that are more RLS friendly and still treat the comorbid problem (see *Chapter 8* and *Chapter 12* for suggestions). Other medical conditions, such as pain from an orthopedic problem (back pain) or neuropathy and anxiety, may trigger increased RLS symptoms and should be investigated then appropriately treated.

Decreasing Iron Levels/Stores

This is often an appropriate time to reassess the patient's serum ferritin level although they should be checked regularly. As iron levels can diminish slowly, this problem may occur unexpectedly and respond to iron therapy. Patients may also have comorbid problems like a bleeding ulcer or gastrointestinal cancer that may be responsible for the decreased iron levels and diagnosing these conditions may be life-saving.

Worsening Due to Tolerance

It is always possible that tolerance to the drugs may develop with time. Usually, an increase in the dose will overcome this problem. However, when doses exceed the recommended ranges, other strategies should be considered. There are varying degrees of cross-tolerance amongst the drugs used for RLS but changing to another medication in the class may resolve the problem.

When tolerance develops to a dopamine agonist, its replacement dopamine agonist may also eventually cause tolerance. Some patient may benefit from rotating these dopamine agonists every few weeks or months to maintain efficacy (see rotation therapy below). Due to a lack of evidence, it is less clear whether this rotation method is suitable for $\alpha2\delta$ ligands.

If the aforementioned techniques do not help, following the algorithm's guidelines as discussed should provide relief.

Worsening Due to Progression of the Disease

RLS tends to be a slowly progressive disease with symptoms worsening over years to decades.[16] Although most patients continue to benefit from small increases in their medication with this disease progression, some may experience more profound worsening of their symptoms that no longer respond to their treatment. Of course, as noted, other reasons for worsening, such as new triggers or low iron levels, should be ruled out.

Once the suggested dose ranges are exceeded, the steps as outlined should be followed. These include a change to another drug in the same class, change to another class of medication including opioids, or combination therapy.

■ Intolerable Side Effects

The approved dopamine agonists and α2δ ligands are typically well tolerated, especially at the lower doses used by RLS patients. However, some patients are sensitive to these drugs and will have trouble tolerating them.

Dopamine Agonists

The most common side effect of the dopamine agonists is nausea, which may often be mitigated by taking the medication with food (however, onset will be delayed by 1 hour). Dizziness and postural hypotension may also occur, especially with the concomitant use of hypertensive medication or if patients become dehydrated. Sleepiness may actually be a beneficial side effect when the medication is taken at bedtime. However, if the drowsiness persists into the morning or if the medication is needed during the daytime, this problem may become disabling. Insomnia is another common side effect that may lead to discontinuation of the medication. If the problem is mild and can be resolved with occasional use of hypnotics, the dopamine agonist can be continued. The most common problem with the rotigotine patch is application site reactions. Rotation of the patch sites helps reduce this problem but if it persists and is significant, use of the patch may have to be stopped.

If any of the more serious but much less common side effects occur (eg, hallucinations, compulsive behavior, or a paradoxical worsening of RLS), the medication must be stopped or reduced and other treatments may need to be considered as per **Figure 10.3**.

α2δ Ligands

The most common side effects of gabapentin enacarbil are dizziness and sedation. These are somewhat dose related and may limit the use of the drug. If this side effect is mild to moderate and not severely affecting the patients, waiting a few weeks will often lead to dissipation of the problem. If the sedation occurs the next day only, the pill can be taken earlier than the suggested 5-6 PM time (as long as it does not cause sedation later in that day well before bedtime), it can be taken without food which should significantly reduce the absorption of the drug or the patient can change to the lower 300-mg renal tablet.

If the more serious but less common class side effects such as DRESS syndrome and suicidal ideation/behavior occur, the drug should be stopped immediately and an alternative therapy (likely not another α2δ ligand) should be considered per **Figure 10.3**.

■ **Augmentation That Is Not Controllable With Additional Earlier Doses of the Drug**

Augmentation (see *Chapter 9*) with dopamine agonists may be a mild problem that can treated simply by taking the drug earlier or adding an extra dose earlier in the day.[17,18] However, some patients progress quickly to needing medication very early in the day with a marked increase in the intensity of their symptoms. They often cannot sit for very long due to the increase in RLS symptoms, and increasing the dose of their dopaminergic drug only relieves the problem temporarily. As stressed above, keeping the dopamine agonist dose as low as possible may prevent worsening augmentation. In addition, checking serum ferritin levels and treating with supplemental iron therapy may be helpful in avoiding and treating the progression of augmentation.

When RLS continues to worsen despite an escalation in the dopamine agonist dose, it is time to stop the medication and change therapy. Typically, medium- to high-potency opioids can be used to treat the marked exacerbation of RLS symptoms that occurs upon withdrawal of the drug. After several weeks or months, an α2δ ligand may be added if the physician wishes to reduce or eliminate the opioid. For further details on how to treat augmentation, see *Chapter 9*.

Individualized Treatment, Combination Treatment, Drug Holidays, and Rotating Treatment

■ Individualized Treatment

It would be nice if we could classify every patient into one of the treatment categories defined in this chapter. However, patients tend to have unique needs and problems that often are not solved by the recommendations in the described therapeutic plans. One of the keys to treating RLS patients is to be flexible. Often several different drugs, doses, and combinations need to be tried. At times, it may be quite frustrating to deal with this condition. However, with patience and guided trial and error, most RLS sufferers can achieve relief from even very bothersome symptoms.

Therapy with just one drug usually works well for most patients with mild-to-moderate RLS. However, many may still have special situations that require additional or different therapy as discussed below in combination therapy. For difficult cases, also consider drug holidays and rotating drugs.

Remember to treat daytime RLS symptoms. If they occur daily, then one extra earlier dose of a short-acting dopamine agonist or α2δ ligand or even better, a long-acting dopamine agonist (or possibly an extended release α2δ ligand) may be necessary. Add a quick-acting medication, such as L-dopa or an opioid analgesic, for as-needed use if daytime symptoms occur sporadically.

■ Combination Treatment

Patients with severe RLS tend to be more difficult to treat. Dopamine agonists or α2δ ligands alone may not resolve their symptoms. Combining different classes of medication may become necessary. Furthermore, for patients who are sensitive to the side effects of medications, combination therapy allows for lower doses of each medication, which may decrease adverse reactions. Typically, it is best to combine an approved dopamine agonist and α2δ ligand before trying the unapproved drugs.

Adding a hypnotic for sleep can be helpful for many RLS patients as they often suffer from insomnia. Even those with mild intermittent RLS may have insomnia and benefit from such medication. An α2δ ligand may also promote sleep and may help decrease painful RLS and associated neuropathy symptoms. By themselves, α2δ ligands usually are not as potent as the dopamine agonists or opioid analgesics for relieving severe RLS symptoms, but they may work well in combination with other drugs. However, it is often necessary to add an opioid to get control of the symptoms in patients with very severe and refractory disease. As discussed earlier in the section on refractory RLS, opioids should not be withheld when needed and can be very effective and safe for long-term therapy.

If symptoms are still not resolved after adding or trying all of the traditionally accepted RLS drugs earlier, think about adding a drug from the other RLS drug list (see *Chapter 9*). Being flexible may help solve difficult-to-treat RLS cases.

Milder cases also benefit from combination therapy. Although most of these patients do well with a daily evening dose of a dopamine agonist or α2δ ligand, many situations require additional therapy. Unexpected sedentary situations (ie, a movie or a trip), unanticipated acute exacerbations of RLS, or just forgetting to take the medication on time all require quick treatment. Since the dopamine agonists require 1 to 3 hours until onset and the α2δ ligands require a few hours, a short-acting, quick-onset drug should be given to most patients for acute treatment. Typically, an opioid analgesic or L-dopa works best in these situations. Therefore, RLS patients should have a prescription for an opioid analgesic or L-dopa and keep a small supply in their car, purse, office, or other places where they can be easily accessed when needed.

■ Drug Holidays

The concept of drug holidays is associated with medications that may cause tolerance. Although the mechanism of tolerance is not well understood, it is thought to be a receptor phenomenon in which continued binding by a medication causes down-regulation of the receptor, which results in a decreased response to that medication. Stopping the medication for a short time for a drug holiday often restores the receptor's full functionality and thus re-establishes the medication's full potency.

RLS medications associated with tolerance include the dopamine agonists, opioids, $\alpha2\delta$ ligands (based on limited clinical experience) and sedative hypnotics. When tolerance is suspected for any of these classes, it is often better to stop the medication for a few weeks instead of potentially worsening the problem by increasing the dose. When restarting the medication, using lower doses may be helpful to prevent the recurrence of tolerance.

Another strategy to prevent the recurrence of tolerance may be to take the medication on an intermittent basis, such as 3 to 4 days per week (often using the drug every other day). Since tolerance may occur from the constant bombardment of the drug's receptor, intermittent use may give the receptor frequent "mini" drug holidays, thus preventing tolerance from occurring. In fact, the intermittent medical use of opioids and benzodiazepines has not been shown to cause tolerance.

■ Rotating Treatment

The concept of rotating treatment shares the same mechanism as drug holidays. Both strategies are helpful for medications that may cause tolerance. When tolerance occurs with a dopamine agonist, changing to another may resolve the problem as cross-tolerance does not usually occur. However, some patients do develop tolerance to the replacement drug, at which point another one can be tried. It is not rare for some patients to rotate two dopamine agonists every few months as they become less active. Some RLS patients have kept their treatment regimen potent for over a decade by rotating the agents.

Since cross-tolerance occurs mostly with benzodiazepines and opioids, this technique of rotating them within their class would not work. However, some patients rotate the benzodiazepines or opioids with other drugs. This really is just simulating intermittent use of the drug as described for the mini drug holiday. The benzodiazepines can even be rotated with the opioids. They can be used on alternate days or 3 to 4 days in a row. While this rotation technique has never been formally studied, it may be considered for patients who have had problems with tolerance.

Referrals—When and to Whom?

When should you refer your RLS patient? The answer may differ depending upon the knowledge and comfort level of each physician. RLS is a disorder that should be diagnosed and treated by every primary care physician (PCP) as with other commonly occurring diseases, such as asthma or diabetes. A small percentage of patients with these common diseases are referred to specialists when they are refractory to traditional therapy. As such, almost all patients with intermittent and daily RLS symptoms should be easily handled by their PCP.

Refractory patients may be somewhat more difficult. However, with the help of this chapter, PCPs may find that they can treat many of these cases. Treatment may require learning how to prescribe and maintain unfamiliar medications, but this task should be made easier by referring to the guidelines and detailed information in *Chapter 9*. As opioids are often required, many physicians may not be comfortable prescribing them for daily, long-term use. Referrals to specialists should be made when, despite reading the guidelines and information available for treating such patients, the physician feels unable or uncomfortable doing so.

As each physician treats more and more RLS patients, they may slowly feel more at ease treating the more complicated cases. Even with the benefit of this book, a physician must feel competent and comfortable in prescribing the recommended medications. When in doubt, it is better to refer the patient to a specialist and learn from the specialist. After seeing how the specialist treats these refractory patients, the PCP may gain sufficient knowledge and familiarity to treat these patients on their own.

To whom do you refer your patient? Unfortunately, no doctors are officially labeled as RLS specialists. However, there are many doctors who have spent years treating and doing research on RLS patients. Typically, neurologists, especially those who specialize in movement disorders, tend to have the necessary expertise for treating patients with difficult to treat RLS. They use all of the typical RLS medications, often in much higher doses, to treat Parkinson's disease, epilepsy, neuropathy, and other neurologic disorders. Sleep-disorder specialists often see and treat numerous RLS patients, and most should have considerable expertise in this area, whatever their original speciality (internal medicine, psychiatry, neurology, or other). Many PCPs have taken an interest in RLS and have become proficient treating even the advanced cases.

However, the best way to ensure that the local neurologist, sleep specialist, or PCP with an interest in RLS is capable of treating these difficult, refractory cases is to talk directly with them. If they do acknowledge their expertise in RLS, you will be able to confirm their abilities by seeing how successfully they treat your patients.

REFERENCES

1. Hening WA. Restless legs syndrome: diagnosis and treatment. *Hosp Med.* 1997;33:54-56, 61-66, 68.

2. Silber MH. Restless legs syndrome. *Mayo Clin Proc.* 1997;72: 261-264.

3. Chesson A Jr, Wise M, Davila D, et al. Practice parameters for the treatment of restless legs syndrome and periodic limb movement disorder. An American Academy of Sleep Medicine Report. Standards of Practice Committee of the American Academy of Sleep Medicine. *Sleep.* 1999;22:961-968.

4. Earley CJ. Clinical practice. Restless legs syndrome. *N Engl J Med.* 2003;348:2103-2109.

5. Silber MH, Ehrenberg BL, Allen RP, et al; Medical Advisory Board of the Restless Legs Syndrome Foundation. An algorithm for the management of restless legs syndrome. *Mayo Clin Proc.* 2004;79:916-922.

6. Lesage S, Hening WA. The restless legs syndrome and periodic limb movement disorder: a review of management. *Semin Neurol.* 2004;24:249-259.

7. Hening WA. Current guidelines and standards of practice for restless legs syndrome. *Am J Med.* 2007;120(1 suppl 1):s22-s27.

8. Garcia-Borreguero D, Stillman P, Benes H, et al. Algorithms for the diagnosis and treatment of restless legs syndrome in primary care. *BMC Neurol.* 2011;11:28.

9. Aukerman MM, Aukerman D, Bayard M, Tudiver F, Thorp L, Bailey B. Exercise and restless legs syndrome: a randomized controlled trial. *J Am Board Fam Med.* 2006;19:487-493.

10. Sun ER, Chen CA, Ho G, Earley CJ, Allen RP. Iron and the restless legs syndrome. *Sleep.* 1998;21:371-377.

11. O'Keeffe ST, Gavin K, Lavan JN. Iron status and restless legs syndrome in the elderly. *Age Ageing.* 1994;23:200-203.

12. Garcia-Borreguero D, Allen RP, Kohnen R. Summary of the recommendations for the long-term treatment of RLS/WED from an IRLSSG Task Force. International Restless Legs Syndrome Study Group Web site. http://irlssg.org/summary. Accessed March 13, 2013.

13. Tzonova D, Larrosa O, Calvo E, et al. Breakthrough symptoms during the daytime in patients with restless legs syndrome (Willis-Ekbom disease). *Sleep Med.* 2012;13(2):151-155.

14. Allen RP, Picchietti D, Hening WA, Trenkwalder C, Walters AS, Montplaisi J; Restless Legs Syndrome Diagnosis and Epidemiology workshop at the National Institutes of Health; International Restless Legs Syndrome Study Group. Restless legs syndrome: diagnostic criteria, special considerations, and epidemiology. A report from the restless legs syndrome diagnosis and epidemiology workshop at the National Institutes of Health. *Sleep Med.* 2003;4:101-119.

15. Aurora RN, Kristo DA, Bista SR, et al. The treatment of restless legs syndrome and periodic limb movement disorder in adults-an update for 2012: practice parameters with an evidence-based systematic review and meta-analysis: an American Academy of Sleep Medicine Clinical Practice Guideline. *Sleep.* 2012;35(8):1039-1062.

16. Hening W, Walters AS, Allen RP, Montplaisir J, Myers A, Ferini-Strambi L. Impact, diagnosis and treatment of restless legs syndrome (RLS) in a primary care population: the REST (RLS epidemiology, symptoms, and treatment) primary care study. *Sleep Med.* 2004;5:237-246.

17. Silber MH, Girish M, Izurieta R. Pramipexole in the management of restless legs syndrome: an extended study. *Sleep.* 2003; 26(7):819-821.

18. Winkelman JW, Johnston L. Augmentation and tolerance with long-term pramipexole treatment of restless legs syndrome (RLS). *Sleep Med.* 2004;5(1):9-14.

10

11 Special Considerations

There are different groups of patients and situations that require special consideration. These groups include children and adolescents, the elderly, women who are pregnant or breastfeeding, surgical patients, and those patients with secondary RLS or PLMD. Treatment plans have to be modified to avoid causing problems by not accommodating the special needs of these groups or situations.

Secondary RLS

Secondary RLS is defined as RLS that occurs due to another underlying medical condition. Typically, this includes three main conditions:
- Iron deficiency
- Renal failure
- Pregnancy.

As discussed in *Chapter 3*, several other neurologic and endocrine disorders may also be causes of secondary RLS. One of the goals for treating secondary RLS is to treat or resolve the primary condition. If that is not possible, the RLS is often treated similarly to idiopathic RLS, as long as the medications do not interfere with the underlying disorder.

■ Iron Deficiency With or Without Anemia

Iron deficiency as a cause of RLS was first noted by Nils Brage Norlander in 1953.[1] He found in an open-label study that large doses of intravenous iron provided 21 of 22 patients complete relief of their RLS for several months. O'Keeffe and colleagues next examined iron as therapy for RLS in an unblinded study in 1993 and found that oral iron therapy with ferrous sulfate 200 mg three times daily improved

RLS symptoms.[2,3] They also discovered that the pre-treatment level of serum ferritin determined whether patients responded to iron. Those patients with levels <18 mcg/L responded best, those whose levels were between 18 and 45 mcg/L responded but not as well as the lower ferritin group, and those patients with levels >45 mcg/L responded minimally. Another study performed by the Johns Hopkins group found that lower serum ferritin levels correlated with greater RLS severity, and all but one patient with severe RLS had serum ferritin levels <50 mcg/L.[4]

These studies have led us to check serum ferritin levels on RLS patients and treat them if the levels are <50 mcg/L. It should be noted that most laboratories report levels >10-20 mcg/L as normal. Additionally, many patients with iron deficiency do not have anemia[5] and the two studies discussed above did not find any significant correlation with serum iron levels and RLS severity.[2-4] Therefore, even when RLS patients present with no signs of iron deficiency (eg, anemia or low serum iron levels), a serum ferritin level should still be assessed. Note that ferritin is an acute-phase reactant, so it must be rechecked as it may be falsely elevated if the patient has any acute illness when drawn.

When serum ferritin levels are <50 mcg/L (even with a normal hemoglobin and serum iron level), oral iron supplementation is generally initiated with 325 mg ferrous sulfate, fumarate, or gluconate (65 mg of elemental iron) up to three times per day on an empty stomach with 100 to 200 mg of vitamin C, as tolerated. Many patients cannot tolerate oral iron, most often because of GI side effects. However, for those who can tolerate oral iron, the goal is to raise serum ferritin levels >50 mcg/L. The serum ferritin level should be monitored periodically to avoid iron overload (ferritin levels >200 mcg/L). Iron repletion is to be avoided in patients with hemochromatosis, who are prone to accumulate toxic levels of iron. They may have a normal ferritin level, but their percent saturation will be notably elevated.

For those RLS patients with significant anemia that cannot be corrected with oral iron, intravenous iron dextran may be a reasonable choice as it has been demonstrated to improve symptoms markedly.[6,7] For other RLS patients, this therapy is still too experimental to be applied to those without resistant anemia.

■ Uremia

Secondary RLS in ESRD with uremia is common, with reported prevalence of up to 83%.[8,9] This can be a major clinical issue for ESRD patients who must sit for several hours a few times per week in their dialysis unit, despite the urge to move because of their secondary RLS. It has also been found that RLS may lower the quality of life and shorten survival in dialysis patients.[10] Clearly, it is important to treat RLS in these patients and it should not be overlooked.

As described in *Chapter 9*, there is ample evidence for improvement of the secondary RLS associated with ESRD through kidney transplantation.[11,12] However, this option is not available to most uremic patients and dialysis does not improve RLS symptoms. Therefore, these patients are treated somewhat similarly to those with idiopathic RLS, taking into consideration the interaction of their renal failure. In fact, most of the suggestions in the algorithm for managing daily RLS (see *Chapter 10*), with some exceptions, may be followed for this group.

Nonpharmacologic Therapy

The steps of the nonpharmacologic therapies[13] outlined in *Chapter 8* and *Chapter 9* apply similarly to uremic patients. This group tends to be more anemic so iron and erythropoietin therapy may be helpful. One study showed temporary benefits (4 weeks) from high-dose IV iron dextran treatment[14] while other studies demonstrated improvement with erythropoietin.[15,16]

Dopaminergic Drugs

Just as with daily idiopathic RLS, dopaminergic drugs are considered the drugs of choice for uremic

RLS.[8] L-dopa has been studied in uremic patients[17-20] and was found to be effective. However, other studies found that gabapentin[20] and ropinirole[21] were more effective than L-dopa for uremic patients. L-dopa may be used at the same doses as for primary RLS but similarly should be reserved for intermittent use (eg, just before dialysis a few times per week) to avoid the high risk of augmentation.

The dopamine agonists are among the most commonly used drugs for significant daily uremic RLS symptoms. Pergolide,[22] pramipexole,[23,24] and ropinirole[25] have been studied and found to be effective for uremic RLS. Ropinirole for uremic RLS can be used exactly as for primary RLS, as it is metabolized in the liver and not excreted through the kidneys. Pergolide and pramipexole are both excreted through the kidneys so should be titrated more slowly and their maximum dose should be limited (0.75 mg for pramipexole). Just as for primary RLS, the ergot-derived dopamine agonists (pergolide, cabergoline, etc), due to their fibrotic side effects, should be considered only when the non-ergot ones are not helpful.

Gabapentin

Two studies have demonstrated the benefits of gabapentin for uremic patients with RLS.[20,26] The drug was found to be more effective than L-dopa in this group and improved sleep, likely due to its sedative properties. Side effects were similar to those in treatment of primary RLS patients, although there is a report of two uremic patients developing myopathy.[27]

This drug is a reasonable alternative to the dopamine agonists. Due to its renal excretion, gabapentin should be given in a reduced dose of 100 to 300 mg after each dialysis.

Opioids

There are no studies on the use of opioids and uremic RLS. Although they may be as effective as for patients with primary RLS, they should be used with caution in ESRD patients since their active metabolites, which normally are excreted by the kidneys, will accumulate.

Benzodiazepines

The first and only study on the use of a benzodiazepine for uremic RLS was in a 1981 report on the benefits of clonazepam 0.5 mg in two split evening doses.[28] The authors found in this open trial that 14 of 15 uremic patients responded to 1 to 2 mg clonazepam daily, but that diazepam did not suppress the symptoms of RLS.

It is likely that the benefits of clonazepam are related to its improvement of insomnia. Similar to those with primary RLS, shorter-acting benzodiazepines or nonbenzodiazepines may be as effective and induce less daytime drowsiness.

■ Other Secondary RLS Conditions

As noted in *Chapter 3*, several other neurologic and endocrine disorders may also be causes of secondary RLS. For the most part, RLS that occurs in association with these conditions is treated similarly to primary RLS. However, for RLS associated with painful neuropathies, anticonvulsants, such as gabapentin or pregabalin,[29] may be more appropriate since they also treat the discomfort from the underlying neurologic disorder. In Parkinson's disease, the schedule of dopaminergic medications can be rearranged to facilitate treating RLS, but in most cases, it will be necessary to use the nondopaminergic medications (eg, anticonvulsants or opioids) to treat RLS.

As with uremia and iron deficiency, treating the underlying disorder may possibly benefit the secondary RLS symptoms. There is one report of a case of RLS that was associated with hyperparathyroidism with hypercalcemia that completely resolved after parathyroidectomy.[30] However, few reports reveal that treating other conditions improves secondary RLS.

About 0.5% of children and 1% of adolescents suffer from RLS. Similar to the algorithm for treating adults, management should begin with nonpharmacologic therapy.[13] When possible, drugs that could potentially worsen RLS (sedating antihistamines, antinausea drugs, antidepressants, etc) should be avoided. Total caffeine restriction (including dietary items, such as chocolate) is suggested due to its effect on RLS and sleep.

Proper sleep hygiene may be very helpful for children. Iron therapy may also be beneficial and as noted with adults, serum ferritin levels should be evaluated. However, there are no guidelines for iron supplementation in children, so physicians should prescribe iron cautiously. The use of lower doses of iron, such as those available with multivitamins containing iron, may be a gentler alternative for treating younger children.

There are no guidelines for treating RLS in children with pharmacologic therapies, as several practice-standards articles have not found sufficient evidence to make any recommendations.[31-33] Children should only be treated with medication when RLS symptoms are severe enough to warrant therapy. Except for clonazepam, which is approved in children for treating seizures, all of the effective drugs are only approved in adults so their use is completely off label.

Due to their generally well-tolerated use in children with ADHD, clonidine and clonazepam have been used frequently in children with RLS. However, as newer drugs are now available, these older medications are prescribed much less often. L-dopa containing drugs have also been used with some success and are well tolerated,[34] but due to concerns of augmentation, they are used much less frequently in all age groups.

Currently, most specialists who treat children for RLS are using the dopamine agonists, ropinirole, and pramipexole. A case study on the treatment of ADHD with ropinirole showed improvement of both ADHD and RLS symptoms in one child, and no adverse events were observed.[35] Studies of pramipexole for treating childhood RLS have yet to be published but one study found it to be well tolerated and effective for PLM in six prepubescent children,[36] while similar results were found when treating two prepubescent children for night terrors and sleepwalking.[37] Both of these drugs should be used at their lowest possible dose (cutting the tablets in half may be reasonable) and increased very slowly.

Pregnant and Breast-Feeding Women

Treating RLS in pregnant and breast-feeding women is often challenging due to the paucity of drugs that are safe in these groups. Care must be taken not to harm the fetus or child. Despite restrictions, there is adequate and safe therapy for these special populations.

■ Pregnant Women

As outlined in *Chapter 3*, RLS is common in pregnant women, especially in the second and third trimesters. RLS symptoms, which can be mild to severe, are superimposed upon the typical discomforts and problems that occur during pregnancy. At times, the disruption of sleep and added discomfort can be almost too much for some women to bear, even though symptoms usually remit within hours to days after delivery.[38]

Treatment begins with nonpharmacologic therapy similar to that for primary RLS. Serum ferritin levels are often decreased during pregnancy, but there are no studies showing benefit from treating with iron and one study revealed no benefit from iron therapy.[39] Another study that looked at iron and ferritin, folic acid, and vitamin B_{12} levels found that only low serum folic acid levels best correlated with RLS.[38] However, most women now take multivitamins that contain sufficient folic acid to avoid fetal neural tube defects. Nevertheless, physicians should check serum iron, ferritin, and folic acid levels in pregnant patients and treat them, if necessary, before starting drug therapy.

The use of medications should be reserved for very severe cases where the sleep disruption itself may cause prematurity and difficult delivery.[40] However, currently all of the guideline articles,[31,32] including the most current European Federation of Neurological Sciences article on the management of RLS,[33] state that there is insufficient evidence to make any treatment recommendations for RLS during pregnancy. Therefore, the following treatment suggestions are based on practical expert experience treating pregnant women with the few available reasonably safe drugs. When possible, drug use should be limited to the third trimester.

Medication should be chosen according to the Pregnancy Risk Categories outlined in **Table 11.1**. Since there are no safe Category A medications for RLS, the mildly risky Category B drugs are used. Pergolide is no longer available in the United States and cabergoline is expensive. The other effective dopamine agonists are otherwise Category C drugs and should be avoided unless absolutely necessary.

Therefore, most RLS specialists prescribe opioids when necessary. Typically, low-dose methadone or oxycodone is preferred. Some experts prefer methadone since its use in high doses for pregnant addicts has already extensively been reported in the literature, including reasonable outcomes except for neonatal abstinence syndrome and prematurity.[41-43] Opioids must be discontinued late in the pregnancy, as they have been associated with neonatal withdrawal syndrome and respiratory depression.

■ Women Who Are Breast-feeding

Treating women who are breast-feeding their children presents difficulties, as many of the medications pass into the breast milk and may adversely affect the child. This includes gabapentin and other anticonvul-

TABLE 11.1 — FDA Risk Categories for RLS Drugs for Use in Pregnant Patients

Risk Category	Drug
A	None
B	Cabergoline, pergolide (but limited data), zolpidem, methadone (low-dose), oxycodone (short-term use)
C	Pramipexole, ropinirole, rotigotine, lel-evodopa, clonidine, zaleplon, eszopiclone, carbamazepine, gabapentin, propoxyphene, codeine, hydrocodone (all for short-term use), fentanyl, hydromorphone, morphine, demerol, levorphanol, tramadol
D	Alprazolam, clonazepam and most benzodiazepine sedatives; propoxyphene, codeine, hydrocodone, oxycodone (all for long-term use), methadone (higher doses)
X	Temazepam

Category A drugs have been tested and are considered completely safe in pregnancy; Categories B through D drugs represent degrees of danger and known teratogenicity, while Category X drugs are contraindicated in pregnancy.

11

sants, benzodiazepines, nonbenzodiazepine sleeping pills, most opioids (some have not been studied well enough for use in women who are breast-feeding), and tramadol. Methadone is considered reasonably safe in breast-feeding women due to its passing only minimally into breast milk. However, before prescribing methadone for severe RLS symptoms in this group, it might be more prudent to have them stop breast-feeding first.

Dopamine agonists cannot be used in nursing mothers as they decrease prolactin levels that in turn decrease breast milk production.

The Elderly

The elderly represent a very large group of RLS patients. According to the REST General Population

Study, 64% of RLS sufferers were ≥50 years of age, with the peak prevalence increasing until age 79.[44]

The key issue with treating RLS in the elderly is their increased sensitivity and decreased ability to metabolize drugs. They often take multiple other medications, raising the risk for adverse drug interactions. As such, it is often wise to start with low doses (even ½ of the lowest-dose pills) and dose titration should be slower. The algorithm for the management of RLS[13] should be followed for this age group; however, opioids and hypnotics should be used more carefully as they may have increased adverse effects, such as falling.[45]

Another concern is that of secondary RLS since it has been found in >70% of those who have their RLS onset after age 65.[46] This group has been demonstrated to have faster progression of their disease, lower ferritin levels, and increased problems with neuropathy.[46,47] Serum ferritin levels <50 mcg/L were found in 58% of those with onset at >64 years of age compared with 22% of those with onset before age 50 years.[46] Therefore, new-onset RLS in the elderly should warrant a serum ferritin level test, and treatment with iron is suggested if it is <50 mcg/L.

Patients Undergoing Surgery or Outpatient Procedures

Surgical and outpatient procedures can be especially challenging for RLS patients and their physicians. Patients may have trouble staying still when at rest and PLM may cause problems with surgery or procedures. With proper care and knowledge, patients can be made comfortable throughout these procedures and problems are easily avoided.

■ Surgery

PLM is common in RLS patients and can occur during surgical procedures, even with spinal anesthesia.[48-52] This can make surgery very risky and thus needs to be addressed. Usually, this can be resolved by the administration of an opioid (morphine) into the epidural or intrathecal space. Parenteral apomorphine is another alternative.

Medications that tend to exacerbate RLS are commonly used before and after surgery (especially antinausea drugs) and should be avoided as noted in *Chapter 8*. It is easy to choose a more RLS-friendly substitute that will not worsen the RLS symptoms.

For patients undergoing major surgical procedures, especially orthopedic ones, the chief concern is postoperative RLS symptoms caused by bed rest. Typically, this is not as much of a concern in the immediate postoperative period since opioids are used to treat the postsurgical pain. However, when the opioids are withdrawn, RLS symptoms quickly worsen, especially when patients remain somewhat immobilized. RLS medications need to be restarted as soon as patients can take oral medications. If they cannot take oral medications or if those drugs do not fully treat their RLS symptoms, parenteral opioids can be given. An alternative might be transdermal formulations of RLS medications.

Patients who develop RLS symptoms while under local anesthesia respond quickly to parenteral opioids or apomorphine. PLM may also improve with opioids but could do better with apomorphine.

■ **Outpatient Procedures**

Typically, MRI scans, CT scans, EEG/EMG tests, and many other outpatient procedures require patients to rest quietly for prolonged periods. Without proper treatment, this can be impossible for many RLS sufferers. However, pretreating with a dopamine agonist (1 to 3 hours before), L-dopa, or an opioid (30 to 60 minutes before) will usually prevent RLS symptoms or PLM from interrupting the procedure. As these procedures often provoke increased anxiety, a sedative may be added to one of the above drugs if necessary.

If RLS symptoms or PLM occur unexpectedly while the procedure is in progress, parenteral opioids

11

or apomorphine should relieve them effectively and quickly.

Periodic Limb Movement Disorder

Over the past several years, whether or not to treat PLMD has become a very controversial issue. The sleep-specialty community is so divided that two pro and con debates among experts have been published on whether PLM should even be monitored in sleep studies[53,54] and whether PLM are associated with disturbed sleep and should be treated.[55,56]

The basis of this debate is that no study has demonstrated that PLM cause increased sleepiness or insomnia or that any benefit is derived from treating them. In fact, several studies have found that PLM may not be associated with insomnia, hypersomnia, waking up refreshed in the morning, the patient's perception of sleep quality, increased sleepiness on Multiple Sleep Latency Test (MSLT) testing, or by subjective sleepiness scales.[57-59] However, recent studies have found that periodic limb movements in sleep (PLMS) transiently increase the heart rate by 7 to 10 beats/minute[60] and, more importantly, transiently increase blood pressure (an average of 11 mm diastolic, 22 mm systolic [and as much as 40 mm systolic])[61,62] which have been associated with vascular and cardiac damage.[63-65]

So how do we manage patients with PLM? This can be best done by dividing them into different categories. The first category is patients who come in because their bed partner complains about being kicked throughout the night and demands that something be done to resolve the situation. Typically, these patients are among the most motivated of people with PLM who seek medical attention. If the person with PLM has no complaints of insomnia or hypersomnia, then RLS experts are divided on whether it is appropriate to treat them with medication (despite their demands for drug treatment). The simplest solution is for the couple to purchase twin-size beds and separate them by an inch at bedtime or invest in a king-size bed with a visco-elastic mattress (such as a TempurPedic). This should prevent the PLM kicks from disrupting the harmony of the relationship while allowing the couple to share a bed.

The second category of patients consists of those who complain that the PLM are vigorous and frequent enough to prevent their falling asleep or that the movements wake them up and then prevent their falling back to sleep. As these PLM occur while the patient is awake, there is no need to obtain a sleep study to verify the problem. These patients warrant a trial of drug treatment to see if their problem can be relieved pharmacologically.

The third category is comprised of patients who are very sleepy or who have insomnia and are not aware of their PLM other than from reports from their bed partner. Although the PLM may be responsible for their sleep problem, other conditions (eg, narcolepsy, sleep apnea, and REM behavior disorder) are also associated with PLM and need to be ruled out. Therefore, to warrant treatment these patients should have an overnight sleep study to determine that they do not have any other underlying sleep disorders and that the PLM are frequent and associated with arousals. There is also some controversy as to what frequency of PLM is abnormally high. Recent studies in older women (average age of 83 years) found that 52% of them had a PLM Index of >15/hour.[66] Therefore, it is not clear as to how many PLM per hour are necessary to warrant treatment. Most sleep specialists who do believe that PLM should be treated will usually consider treating patients when there are >40-50 PLM/hour associated with arousals (although this may vary considerably as there are no guidelines). If no other medical conditions or reasons can explain the patient's hypersomnia or insomnia, a trial of medication may be warranted to see if it helps the sleep-related complaints.

The last category is those patients who have a sleep study to rule out another condition, such as sleep apnea, and frequent PLM are reported. Similar to the patients above, if they have no other sleep disorder, yet have sleep-related complaints of hypersomnia or insomnia, a trial of drug therapy may be reasonable.

Before treating the patient for PLM pharmacologically, the physician should review the patient's current medications. Typically, antidepressants (especially the SSRIs and SNRIs) increase PLM[67] and if medically appropriate, a change to bupropion (which does not worsen PLM) may be helpful. In addition, physicians should question patients further about RLS symptoms as this is commonly a comorbid condition (>85% of RLS patients have PLM) that can be easily missed. If these patients need treatment for their RLS, those therapies will typically resolve their PLM at the same time.

For treating PLMD, the dopaminergic drugs (L-dopa, pergolide, pramipexole, and ropinirole) are considered effective to reduce the severity of PLM.[68] Most experts who treat RLS and PLMD consider dopamine agonists such as ropinirole and pramipexole to be the most effective treatment for PLMD and one of the best tolerated.

There is also evidence that gabapentin is effective for PLM.[69-71] Opioids help RLS symptoms but there are few studies on their benefits for PLM.[72,73]

Benzodiazepines have been used to treat PLMD, but although some studies show that they decrease PLM,[74-77] most other studies found that they do not decrease the amount of PLM but rather decrease the arousals caused by the PLM and improve sleep quality.[78-82] These studies were done using clonazepam, temazepam, and triazolam, and any of these medications would be a reasonable choice to treat a patient with PLMD, especially if the patient complains about poor sleep quality or insomnia. However, similar to treating RLS, the shorter-acting benzodiazepines or nonbenzodiazepines may be preferred.

REFERENCES

1. Norlander NB. Therapy in restless legs. *Acta Med Scand*. 1953; 145:453-457.

2. O'Keeffe ST, Noel J, Lavan JN. Restless legs syndrome in the elderly. *Postgrad Med J*. 1993;69:701-703.

3. O'Keeffe ST, Gavin K, Lavan JN. Iron status and restless legs syndrome in the elderly. *Age Ageing*. 1994;23(3):200-203.

4. Sun ER, Chen CA, Ho G, Earley CJ, Allen RP. Iron and the restless legs syndrome. *Sleep*. 1998;21:371-377.

5. Looker AC, Dallman PR, Carroll MD, Gunter EW, Johnson CL. Prevalence of iron deficiency in the United States. *JAMA*. 1997;277:973-976.

6. Earley CJ, Heckler D, Allen RP. The treatment of restless legs syndrome with intravenous iron dextran. *Sleep Med*. 2004; 5:231-235.

7. Earley CJ, Heckler D, Allen RP. Repeated IV doses of iron provides effective supplemental treatment of restless legs syndrome. *Sleep Med*. 2005;6:301-305.

8. Kavanagh D, Siddiqui S, Geddes CC. Restless legs syndrome in patients on dialysis. *Am J Kidney Dis*. 2004;43:763-771.

9. Molnar MZ, Novak M, Mucsi I. Management of restless legs syndrome in patients on dialysis. *Drugs*. 2006;66:607-624.

10. Unruh ML, Levey AS, D'Ambrosio C, Fink NE, Powe NR, Meyer KB; Choices for Healthy Outcomes in Caring for End-Stage Renal Disease (CHOICE) Study. Restless legs symptoms among incident dialysis patients: association with lower quality of life and shorter survival. *Am J Kidney Dis*. 2004;43:900-909.

11. Yasuda T, Nishimura A, Katsuki Y, Tsuji Y. Restless legs syndrome treated successfully by kidney transplantation–a case report. *Clin Transpl*. 1986:138.

12. Winkelmann J, Stautner A, Samtleben W, Trenkwalder C. Long-term course of restless legs syndrome in dialysis patients after kidney transplantation. *Mov Disord*. 2002;17:1072-1076.

13. Silber MH, Ehrenberg BL, Allen RP, et al; Medical Advisory Board of the Restless Legs Syndrome Foundation. An algorithm for the management of restless legs syndrome. *Mayo Clin Proc*. 2004;79:916-922.

14. Sloand JA, Shelly MA, Feigin A, Bernstein P, Monk RD. A double-blind, placebo-controlled trial of intravenous iron dextran therapy in patients with ESRD and restless legs syndrome. *Am J Kidney Dis*. 2004;43:663-670.

11

15. Harris DC, Chapman JR, Stewart JH, Lawrence S, Roger SD. Low dose erythropoietin in maintenance haemodialysis: improvement in quality of life and reduction in true cost of haemodialysis. *Aust N Z J Med.* 1991;21:693-700.

16. Benz RL, Pressman MR, Hovick ET, Peterson DD. A preliminary study of the effects of correction of anemia with recombinant human erythropoietin therapy on sleep, sleep disorders, and daytime sleepiness in hemodialysis patients (The SLEEPO study). *Am J Kidney Dis.* 1999;34:1089-1095.

17. Sandyk R, Bernick C, Lee SM, Stern LZ, Iacono RP, Bamford CR. L-dopa in uremic patients with the restless legs syndrome. *Int J Neurosci.* 1987;35:233-235.

18. Wetter TC, Trenkwalder C, Stiasny K, et al. Treatment of idiopathic and uremic restless legs syndrome with L-dopa—a double-blind cross-over study. *Wien Med Wochenschr.* 1995; 145:525-527.

19. Trenkwalder C, Stiasny K, Pollmacher T, et al. L-dopa therapy of uremic and idiopathic restless legs syndrome: a double-blind, crossover trial. *Sleep.* 1995;18:681-688.

20. Micozkadioglu H, Ozdemir FN, Kut A, Sezer S, Saatci U, Haberal M. Gabapentin versus levodopa for the treatment of Restless Legs Syndrome in hemodialysis patients: an open-label study. *Ren Fail.* 2004;26:393-397.

21. Pellecchia MT, Vitale C, Sabatini M, et al. Ropinirole as a treatment of restless legs syndrome in patients on chronic hemodialysis: an open randomized crossover trial versus levodopa sustained release. *Clin Neuropharmacol.* 2004;27:178-181.

22. Pieta J, Millar T, Zacharias J, Fine A, Kryger M. Effect of pergolide on restless legs and leg movements in sleep in uremic patients. *Sleep.* 1998;21:617-622.

23. Miranda M, Fabres L, Kagi M, et al. Treatment of restless legs syndrome in uremic patients undergoing dialysis with pramipexole: preliminary results. *Rev Med Chil.* 2003;131:700-701.

24. Miranda M, Kagi M, Fabres L, et al. Pramipexole for the treatment of uremic restless legs in patients undergoing hemodialysis. *Neurology.* 2004;62:831-832.

25. Pellecchia MT, Vitale C, Sabatini M, et al. Ropinirole as a treatment of restless legs syndrome in patients on chronic hemodialysis: an open randomized crossover trial versus levodopa sustained release. *Clin Neuropharmacol.* 2004;27:178-181.

26. Thorp ML, Morris CD, Bagby SP. A crossover study of gabapentin in treatment of restless legs syndrome among hemodialysis patients. *Am J Kidney Dis.* 2001;38:104-108.

27. Lipson J, Lavoie S, Zimmerman D. Gabapentin-induced myopathy in 2 patients on short daily hemodialysis. *Am J Kidney Dis*. 2005;45:e100-e104.

28. Read DJ, Feest TG, Nassim MA. Clonazepam: effective treatment for restless legs syndrome in uraemia. *Br Med J (Clin Res Ed)*. 1981;283:885-886.

29. Sommer M, Bachmann CG, Liebetanz KM, Schindehutte J, Tings T, Paulus W. Pregabalin in restless legs syndrome with and without neuropathic pain. *Acta Neurol Scand*. 2007;115: 347-350.

30. Lim LL, Dinner D, Tham KW, Siraj E, Shields R Jr. Restless legs syndrome associated with primary hyperparathyroidism. *Sleep Med*. 2005;6:283-285.

31. Chesson AL Jr, Wise M, Davila D, et al. Practice parameters for the treatment of restless legs syndrome and periodic limb movement disorder. An American Academy of Sleep Medicine Report. Standards of Practice Committee of the American Academy of Sleep Medicine. *Sleep*. 1999;22:961-968.

32. Littner MR, Kushida C, Anderson WM, et al. Standards of Practice Committee of the American Academy of Sleep Medicine. Practice parameters for the dopaminergic treatment of restless legs syndrome and periodic limb movement disorder. *Sleep*. 2004;27:557-559.

33. Vignatelli L, Billiard M, Clarenbach P, et al. EFNS Task Force. EFNS guidelines on management of restless legs syndrome and periodic limb movement disorder in sleep. *Eur J Neurol*. 2006;13:1049-1065.

34. Walters AS, Mandelbaum DE, Lewin DS, Kugler S, England SJ, Miller M. Dopaminergic therapy in children with restless legs/periodic limb movements in sleep and ADHD. Dopaminergic Therapy Study Group. *Pediatr Neurol*. 2000;22:182-186.

35. Konofal E, Arnulf I, Lecendreux M, Mouren MC. Ropinirole in a child with attention-deficit hyperactivity disorder and restless legs syndrome. *Pediatr Neurol*. 2005;32:350-351.

36. Martinez S, Guilleminault C. Periodic leg movements in prepubertal children with sleep disturbance. *Dev Med Child Neurol*. 2004;46:765-770.

37. Guilleminault C, Palombini L, Pelayo R, Chervin RD. Sleep-walking and sleep terrors in prepubertal children: what triggers them? *Pediatrics*. 2003;111:e17-e25.

38. Lee KA, Zaffke ME, Baratte-Beebe K. Restless legs syndrome and sleep disturbance during pregnancy: the role of folate and iron. *J Womens Health Gend Based Med*. 2001;10:335-341.

11

39. Manconi M, Govoni V, De Vito A, et al. Restless legs syndrome and pregnancy. *Neurology*. 2004;63:1065-1069.

40. Manconi M, Ferini-Strambi L, Hening WA. Response to Clinical Corners case (Sleep Medicine 6/2: 83-4): Pregnancy associated with daytime sleepiness and nighttime restlessness. *Sleep Med*. 2005;6:477-478.

41. Wang EC. Methadone treatment during pregnancy. *J Obstet Gynecol Neonatal Nurs*. 1999;28:615-622.

42. McCarthy JJ, Leamon MH, Parr MS, Anania B. High-dose methadone maintenance in pregnancy: maternal and neonatal outcomes. *Am J Obstet Gynecol*. 2005;193:606-610.

43. Lejeune C, Simmat-Durand L, Gourarier L, Aubisson S; Groupe d'Etudes Grossesse et Addictions (GEGA). Prospective multicenter observational study of 260 infants born to 259 opiate-dependent mothers on methadone or high-dose buprenophine substitution. *Drug Alcohol Depend*. 2006;82:250-257.

44. Allen RP, Walters AS, Montplaisir J, et al. Restless legs syndrome prevalence and impact: REST general population study. *Arch Intern Med*. 2005;165:1286-1292.

45. Mendelson WB. The use of sedative/hypnotic medication and its correlation with falling down in the hospital. *Sleep*. 1996; 19:698-701.

46. O'Keeffe ST. Secondary causes of restless legs syndrome in older people. *Age Ageing*. 2005;34:349-352.

47. Allen RP, Earley CJ. Defining the phenotype of the restless legs syndrome (RLS) using age-of-symptom-onset. *Sleep Med*. 2000;1:11-19.

48. Shin YK. Restless leg syndrome: unusual cause of agitation under anesthesia. *South Med J*. 1987;80:278-279.

49. Martinez LP, Koza M. Anesthesia-related periodic involuntary movement in an obstetrical patient for cesarean section under epidural anesthesia: a case report. *AANA J*. 1997;65(2):150-153.

50. Moorthy SS, Dierdorf SF. Restless legs during recovery from spinal anesthesia. *Anesth Analg*. 1990;70:337.

51. Watanabe S, Sakai K, Ono Y, Seino H, Naito H. Alternating periodic leg movement induced by spinal anesthesia in an elderly male. *Anesth Analg*. 1987;66:1031-1032.

52. Watanabe S, Ono A, Naito H. Periodic leg movements during either epidural or spinal anesthesia in an elderly man without sleep-related (nocturnal) myoclonus. *Sleep*. 1990;13:262-266.

53. Mahowald MW. Con: assessment of periodic leg movements is not an essential component of an overnight sleep study. *Am J Respir Crit Care Med.* 2001;164:1340-1341.

54. Walters AS. Pro: assessment of periodic leg movements is an essential component of an overnight sleep study. *Am J Respir Crit Care Med.* 2001;164:1339-1340.

55. Mahowald MW. Periodic limb movements are NOT associated with disturbed sleep. *J Clin Sleep Med.* 2007;3:15-17.

56. Hogl B. Periodic limb movements are associated with disturbed sleep. Pro. *J Clin Sleep Med.* 2007;3:12-14.

57. Mendelson WB. Are periodic leg movements associated with clinical sleep disturbance? *Sleep.* 1996;19:219-223.

58. Hilbert J, Mohsenin V. Can periodic limb movement disorder be diagnosed without polysomnography? A case-control study. *Sleep Med.* 2003;4:35-41.

59. Hornyak M, Riemann D, Voderholzer U. Do periodic leg movements influence patients' perception of sleep quality? *Sleep Med.* 2004;5:597-600.

60. Gosselin N, Lanfranchi P, Michaud M, et al. Age and gender effects on heart rate activation associated with periodic leg movements in patients with restless legs syndrome. *Clin Neurophysiol.* 2003;114:2188-2195.

61. Ali NJ, Davies RJ, Fleetham JA, Stradling JR. Periodic movements of the legs during sleep associated with rises in systemic blood pressure. *Sleep.* 1991;14:163-165.

62. Pennestri MH, Montplaisir J, Colombo R, Lavigne G, Lanfranchi PA. Nocturnal blood pressure changes in patients with restless legs syndrome. *Neurology.* 2007;68:1213-1218.

63. Frattola A, Parati G, Cuspidi C, Albini F, Mancia G. Prognostic value of 24-hour blood pressure variability. *J Hypertens.* 1993; 11:1133-1137.

64. Zakopoulos NA, Tsivgoulis G, Barlas G, et al. Time rate of blood pressure variation is associated with increased common carotid artery intima-media thickness. *Hypertension.* 2005;45:505-512.

65. Roman MJ, Pickering TG, Schwartz JE, Pini R, Devereux RB. Relation of blood pressure variability to carotid atherosclerosis and carotid artery and left ventricular hypertrophy. *Arterioscler Thromb Vasc Biol.* 2001;21:1507-1511.

66. Claman DM, Redline S, Blackwell T, et al. Study of Osteoporotic Fratures Research Group. Prevalence and correlates of periodic limb movements in older women. *J Clin Sleep Med.* 2006;2:438-445.

11

67. Yang C, White DP, Winkelman JW. Antidepressants and periodic leg movements of sleep. *Biol Psychiatry*. 2005;58:510-514.

68. Littner MR, Kushida C, Anderson WM, et al. Standards of Practice Committee of the American Academy of Sleep Medicine. Practice parameters for the dopaminergic treatment of restless legs syndrome and periodic limb movement disorder. *Sleep*. 2004;27:557-559.

69. Happe S, Klosch G, Saletu B, Zeitlhofer J. Treatment of idiopathic restless legs syndrome (RLS) with gabapentin. *Neurology*. 2001;57:1717-1719.

70. Garcia-Borreguero D, Larrosa O, de la Llave Y, Verger K, Masramon X, Hernandez G. Treatment of restless legs syndrome with gabapentin: a double-blind, cross-over study. *Neurology*. 2002;59:1573-1579.

71. Happe S, Sauter C, Klosch G, Saletu B, Zeitlhofer J. Gabapentin versus ropinirole in the treatment of idiopathic restless legs syndrome. *Neuropsychobiology*. 2003;48:82-86.

72. Kaplan PW, Allen RP, Buchholz DW, Walters JK. A double-blind, placebo-controlled study of the treatment of periodic limb movements in sleep using carbidopa/levodopa and propoxyphene. *Sleep*. 1993;16:717-723.

73. Walters AS, Wagner ML, Hening WA, et al. Successful treatment of the idiopathic restless legs syndrome in a randomized double-blind trial of oxycodone versus placebo. *Sleep*. 1993;16:327-332.

74. Ohanna N, Peled R, Rubin AH, Zomer J, Lavie P. Periodic leg movements in sleep: effect of clonazepam treatment. *Neurology*. 1985;35:408-411.

75. Peled R, Lavie P. Double-blind evaluation of clonazepam on periodic leg movements in sleep. *J Neurol Neurosurg Psychiatry*. 1987;50:1679-1681.

76. Edinger JD, Fins AI, Sullivan RJ, Marsh GR, Dailey DS, Young M. Comparison of cognitive-behavioral therapy and clonazepam for treating periodic limb movement disorder. *Sleep*. 1996;19:442-444.

77. Horiguchi J, Inami Y, Sasaki A, Nishimatsu O, Sukegawa T. Periodic leg movements in sleep with restless legs syndrome: effect of clonazepam treatment. *Jpn J Psychiatry Neurol*. 1992;46(3):727-732.

78. Mitler MM, Browman CP, Menn SJ, Gujavarty K, Timms RM. Nocturnal myoclonus: treatment efficacy of clonazepam and temazepam. *Sleep*. 1986;9:385-392.

79. Bonnet MH, Arand DL. The use of triazolam in older patients with periodic leg movements, fragmented sleep, and daytime sleepiness. *J Gerontol.* 1990;45:M139-M144.

80. Doghramji K, Browman CP, Gaddy JR, Walsh JK. Triazolam diminishes daytime sleepiness and sleep fragmentation in patients with periodic leg movements in sleep. *J Clin Psychopharmacol.* 1991;11:284-290.

81. Bonnet MH, Arand DL. Chronic use of triazolam in patients with periodic leg movements, fragmented sleep and daytime sleepiness. *Aging (Milano).* 1991;3(4):313-324.

82. Saletu M, Anderer P, Saletu-Zyhlarz G, et al. Restless legs syndrome (RLS) and periodic limb movement disorder (PLMD): acute placebo-controlled sleep laboratory studies with clonazepam. *Eur Neuropsychopharmacol.* 2001;11:153-161.

11

12

RLS and Psychiatric Disorders

As early as the 19th century, Wittmaack observed the co-occurrence of RLS with depression and anxiety, what he termed "anxietus tibiarum," and believed it to be a form of hysteria.[1] Once considered a rare neurologic disorder treated primarily by neurologists, psychiatrists rarely recognized or treated RLS. Recently, however, RLS has become increasingly important in the practice of psychiatry, as several studies have reported a high prevalence of psychiatric comorbidities among RLS sufferers, particularly depression and anxiety.[2] In fact, previously subsumed under Dysomnia Not Otherwise Specified in the fourth edition of the DSM, RLS is expected to be elevated to a full diagnosis in DSM-5.[3] The rationale for the elevation of RLS to its own diagnostic criteria is based on "strong empirical evidence" for the following:

- Significant prevalence of RLS in the general population
- Association of RLS with significant clinical and functional impairment
- Identified and replicated genetic markers for RLS
- Successful treatment response of RLS
- Evidence for a defined pathophysiological basis of RLS.

Underlying the rationale for elevation of RLS as full diagnostic criteria in DSM-5 is the recognition within the psychiatry field that RLS symptoms are often encountered during evaluation of patients with psychiatric symptoms or on psychiatric medications.

The inclusion of RLS in DSM-5 will likely encourage more frequent evaluation of patients with comorbid RLS and psychiatric disorders in both primary care and specialty practice, especially in psychiatry. The purpose of this chapter is to provide an overview on the clinical aspects of managing RLS in this population.

RLS and Depression and/or Anxiety

Epidemiologically, there are several striking similarities between RLS and mood disorders, especially depression. First, both RLS and major depression have similar prevalence rates in the community. Approximately 5% to 10% of the general population has RLS of varying severity,[5] and the lifetime prevalence of major depressive disorder (MDD) in the community is between 5% to 10%.[6] The mean age of onset for both conditions is in the 30s with a wide distribution.[4,6] Another interesting similarity is the female preponderance of 2 to 1 for both RLS and MDD.[5,7] Furthermore, both RLS and mood disorders have a strong genetic contribution to their etiology since multiple studies have confirmed family history as a strong risk factor.[8,9]

Therefore, it is not surprising that previous clinic-based studies reported a high prevalence of comorbidity between RLS and depression or anxiety disorders. Most of these studies relied on simple depression or anxiety rating scales with limited validity and did not have a control group, but their findings have been consistent.[2] Most notably, Winkelmann and colleagues, utilizing a structured psychiatric interview called the Munich-Composite International Diagnostic Interview for DSM-IV, assessed psychopathology among 130 RLS patients and compared the prevalence of MDD and panic disorder with 2265 residents who participated in a community-based study.[10] The results from this study revealed an increased risk for having 12-month anxiety and depressive disorders with particularly strong associations for panic disorder, generalized anxiety disorder, and major depression (**Table 12.1**). This study focused on a clinical population, which likely had relatively severe RLS symptoms, and contrasted it to a select population sample of those with chronic somatic diseases. These results confirmed the high prevalence of depression and anxiety symptoms in RLS patients.

TABLE 12.1 — Increased Risk of Psychiatric Disorders in RLS

Disorder	Increased Risk
Clinic-Based Sample in Germany[1]	
Panic disorder	OR=4.7 (95% CI=2.1-10.1)
Generalized anxiety disorder	OR=3.5 (95% CI=1.7-7.1)
Major depression	OR=2.6 (95% CI=1.5-4.4)
Community-Based Sample in Baltimore, MD[2]	
Panic disorder	OR[a]=12.9 (95% CI=3.6-46.0)
Major depressive disorder	OR[a]=4.7 (95% CI=1.6, 14.5)

Abbreviations: CI, confidence interval; OR, odds ratio.
[a] These are adjusted odds ratios to account for possible confounds.

[1] Winkelmann J, et al. *Sleep Med*. 2003;4:101-109.
[2] Lee HB, et al. *J Neuropsychiatry Clin Neurosci*. 2007;48:167-169.

Several population-based studies have also reported increased rates of anxiety and depression in subjects with RLS.[2] Unlike clinic-based studies, population-based studies do not have a referral bias and have a comparison group drawn from the same population. Among the previous studies, the more recent RLS in Baltimore Epidemiologic Catchment Area (RiBECA) study provided strong evidence for the association between RLS and depression and/or anxiety disorders.[11] In this study, Lee and associates examined the association between RLS and DSM-IV MDD and panic disorder (based on 1071 participants who completed the seven-item RLS Questionnaire and Diagnostic Interview Schedule). The study found strikingly high odds ratios in RLS patients for both diagnoses of DSM-IV MDD and panic disorder in the past 12 months, suggesting a strong association between RLS and the two disorders (**Table 12.1**). Replication of these findings has been recently reported based on the nationwide survey of 6509 Korean adults.[12]

Whether the close association between RLS and depressive symptoms is a by-product of symptomatic overlap remains an unresolved question. Out of the nine symptoms listed for the MDD diagnostic criteria in the DSM-IV, RLS could trigger or exacerbate at least four of these depressive symptoms (**Table 12.2**).[2] On the other hand, according to the RiBECA study, MDD symptoms supposedly unrelated to RLS (**Table 12.2**) are just as common among those with comorbid RLS and MDD.[11] In other words, the association between RLS and MDD may be more than a superficial similarity due to the diagnostic overlap.

The high prevalence of panic disorder in subjects with RLS is even more intriguing as little symptomatic overlap exists between the two conditions.[12,13] Similarly, a high rate of comorbidity with panic dis-

TABLE 12.2 — Overlapping and Distinctive Criteria for Depression With RLS

Depressive Symptoms That Overlap With RLS
- Insomnia or excessive sleepiness
- Decreased concentration, fatigue, or loss of energy
- Psychomotor retardation
- Dysphoric mood

Depressive Symptoms That Do Not Overlap With RLS
- Appetite loss
- Suicidal thoughts
- Low self-esteem
- Anhedonia
- Weight gain or loss

order and MDD is observable in patients with PD, a neurodegenerative disorder primarily involving central dopaminergic tracts.[14] Psychiatric comorbidities of PD can be attributable to direct dopaminergic deficits or interactions between dopaminergic deficits, as well as to the known variable deficits in norepinephrine and serotonin that occur in PD.[15] Little is known about the role of noradrenergic or serotonergic neurotransmission in the pathophysiology of RLS. Future investigations should examine the pathophysiologic overlap between RLS and MDD or panic disorder that frequently co-occurs in the clinic and in the community.

For example, multiple studies have established the role of dopaminergic pathology in RLs.[16] Several studies also support a role for diminished dopaminergic neurotransmission in MDD.[17] In fact, bupropion, which has proven efficacy in the treatment of depression, acts, at least in part, via promoting dopaminergic function.[18] Several clinical trials recently reported a potential role for dopamine agonists (eg, pramipexole), a common RLS treatment choice, for managing treatment-resistant depression or bipolar depression.[19] Two recent studies are also notable in reporting that dopamine agonist treatment of RLS with ropinirole or pramipexole not only improved the RLS symptoms, but also significantly improved depressive symptoms as well.[20,21] Therefore, in RLS patients with mild depressive symptoms, treatment of RLS symptoms first with dopamine agonist might be a reasonable approach. Often, improvement of RLS-related sleep impairment has a positive effect on reducing depressive symptoms along with potential mood elevating quality of dopamine agonist.

RLS and ADHD

Recently, there has been much interest in a potential association between attention-deficit/hyperactivity disorder (ADHD) and RLS as well.[13] Several studies have reported that RLS and PLMS are common in children or adults with ADHD.[22,23] A review in 2005 estimated that up to 44% of subjects with ADHD have been found to have RLS or RLS symptoms, and up to 26% of subjects with RLS have been found to have ADHD or ADHD symptoms.[13] However, the glaring methodologic limitations of the reviewed studies (eg, questionable case ascertainment method for ADHD and RLS and sampling or referral biases); therefore, it is probable that the real estimates of the prevalence of RLS in ADHD and vice versa are more conservative. However, it is still unclear whether sleep disruption due to RLS rather than RLS itself is associated with ADHD-like symptoms of restlessness, overactivity, and inattention. One study compared ADHD symptoms in adults with RLS, normal controls, and controls with insomnia, and reported that ADHD symptoms are more common in patients with RLS than in patients with insomnia or normal controls.[24] However, diurnal symptoms of restlessness and inattentiveness of RLS could be mimicking ADHD symptoms on the rating scale without true attention deficits or hyperactivity.

RLS and Cognition

The few available studies on the impact of RLS on cognition have yielded inconsistent findings. Two previous studies that compared the cognitive functioning of RLS patients to RLS-free control subjects have reported impairment primarily in executive functioning.[25,26] In contrast, Gamaldo and colleagues reported superior performance on letter and category fluency among untreated RLS patients in comparison to controls.[27] Findings from the population-based studies have also been inconsistent. Celle and colleagues[28] found reduced functioning in the Stroop task and verbal fluency while Driver-Dunckley and associates[29] found no difference in cognitive functioning between those with mild RLS vs those without RLS.

Overall, it seems a common sense that RLS severe enough to cause sleep deprivation would lead to cognitive impairment. However, evidence seems to lack whether or not RLS itself has an impact on cognitive performance.

Management of Psychiatric Medications in RLS Patients

Since RLS and psychiatric disorders co-occur frequently, a clinician should give that fact careful consideration when choosing a medication for a psychiatric patient with comorbid RLS. Many psychiatric medications have the potential to affect RLS symptoms. When neuroleptic or antidepressant medications are used to treat psychiatric disorders, it may be difficult to avoid prescribing them. Stopping or reducing them, even when RLS symptoms are clearly exacerbated, should be done with great trepidation due to concerns about worsening the underlying psychiatric disorder. However, other than case series studies or anecdotal reports, few studies have examined the direct effects of psychiatric medications on RLS symptoms, although several have examined the effect of these medications on the severity of periodic limb movements in sleep (PLMS). Since PLMS occur in at least 80% of RLS patients and correlate with RLS severity, the effects of psychiatric medication on PLMS could be used to infer the effect of psychiatric medicine on RLS as well. Psychoactive medications that are more compatible with RLS are shown in **Table 12**.3.

■ **RLS and Neuroleptic Medications**

Typical neuroleptic medications and newer atypical neuroleptic medications are often used to treat psychiatric conditions such as schizophrenia, bipolar disorders, and treatment-resistant depression. Neuroleptic medications may worsen RLS as they decrease dopamine neurotransmission. In fact, their common side effects include akathisia, a condition that shares many clinical features with RLS. Even common antiemetics (eg, metoclopramide, promethazine, and prochlorperazine) also exacerbate RLS symptoms

TABLE 12.3 — Psychoactive Medications That Are More Compatible With RLS

Medication	Comments
Alternative for Neuroleptics	
Aripiprazole	Functions as a partial agonist at the dopamine D_2 receptor; some anecdotal claims have been made that it may help RLS, but studies are necessary to confirm this benefit
Alternatives for Antidepressants	
Bupropion	A weak dopamine reuptake inhibitor that may possibly help RLS symptoms,[1] and rarely worsens RLS[2]
Trazodone	This drug does not seem to affect RLS and may improve sleep
Desipramine	Although TCAs tend to worsen RLS, the secondary amines, desipramine, protriptyline, and nortriptyline have less serotonergic effects and may be safer for RLS patients
Reboxetine	A selective noradrenergic thought to be neutral for RLS; although widely available, it is not approved in the United States
Nefazodone	This SNRI drug appears to have less serotonin effect than the others; not used very often due to its rare (1/300,000) side effect of liver failure

[1] Kim SW, et al. *Clin Neuropharmacol.* 2005;28:298-301.

[2] Picchietti D, et al. *Sleep.* 2005;28:891-898.

because of their dopamine receptor–blocking property. Newer atypical antipsychotics are less likely to exacerbate PLMS because of their lower binding affinity for the dopamine D_2 receptor, but three reports of initiation or exacerbation of RLS-like symptoms by risperidone, olanzapine, and quetiapine exist.[30-32] There are other case reports in the medical literature that describe the onset of RLS with clozapine[32] and pimozide.[33]

Although there have been no formal studies on these drugs to validate their effect on RLS, many RLS patients have reported worsening symptoms while taking them. Aripiprazole, a partial dopamine agonist, theoretically might have a favorable effect on RLS symptoms, but no systematic study is available on this issue. When neuroleptic medications are used to treat psychotic disorders, it may be difficult to avoid prescribing them unless their psychiatric symptoms are carefully monitored by a psychiatrist. Stopping or reducing them, even when RLS symptoms are clearly exacerbated, should be done with great trepidation due to potential impact on the underlying psychiatric disorder.

■ **RLS and Antidepressants**

There are many case reports of worsening RLS while on many of the selective serotonin reuptake inhibitors (SSRIs), serotonin-norepinephrine reuptake inhibitors (SNRIs), and tricyclics (TCAs). The mechanism of antidepressant, particularly SSRIs, SNRIs, and TCAs, worsening RLS is not fully understood as they do not directly block dopamine.[34] It is thought that the increase in serotonin produced by this class of drugs may exacerbate RLS by serotonergically mediated inhibition of dopaminergic neurotransmission, which may also explain why they cause akathisia.[34] Additionally, these drugs are known to increase PLM,[35] which are thought to be caused by mechanisms similar to RLS.

However, there are no controlled studies validating the link between antidepressant drugs used to treat depression and anxiety and worsening RLS symptoms. Although various TCAs and SSRIs have been suggested to exacerbate PLMS, it is unknown what specific mechanisms exacerbate PLMS. Systematic studies have reported higher PLMS associated with TCAs, SSRIs, and venlafaxine.[35-37] Anecdotal reports of SSRIs (eg, fluoxetine, paroxetine, citalopram, and sertraline) and venlafaxine exacerbating RLS also exist.[38-42]

There are no case reports in the literature about the effect of the TCAs and RLS. However, TCAs (amitriptyline, clomipramine, doxepin, imipramine, trimipramine) increase levels of serotonin similar to the SSRI medications. Anecdotal reports from patients on TCAs have supported their negative effects on RLS. Additionally, increased PLM with this class of medication has been reported.[35] Although there are no reported cases of duloxetine worsening RLS at the moment, SNRIs such as duloxetine and venlafaxine increase levels of serotonin enough that they could potentially exacerbate RLS symptoms. In addition, venlafaxine has been shown to cause as much of an increase in PLM as do the SSRIs.[36] Therefore, among RLS patients and experts, it is commonly believed that SSRIs, SNRIs, and TCAs exacerbate RLS symptoms.

Contradicting these reports are two retrospective studies that report improvement of RLS symptoms while on SSRIs.[43,44] One study reviewed 113 consecutive patients attending a hospital-based clinic who had been prescribed SSRIs (sertraline, paroxetine, or fluoxetine) for depression and found that majority of patients (65%) experienced improvement of their pre-existing RLS symptoms with their SSRI treatment.[43] Another study reviewed 200 consecutive patients presenting for the evaluation of sleep-initiation insomnia at a sleep-disorders center and did not find any link between antidepressant medication and RLS.[44] However, the generalizability of these studies may be limited due to the retrospective design and informal, self-report–based assessment of RLS symptoms. However, it underscores the fact that the role of SSRI/SNRI/TCA in the treatment of RLS patients with a mood disorder remains somewhat unclear despite commonly held belief that these antidepressants are "RLS-unfriendly."

The effect of mirtazapine, a heterocyclic antidepressant, on RLS symptoms remains unclear. Often, mirtazapine, a sedating antidepressant, is prescribed to treat insomnia symptoms of depression. However, case reports have reported worsening of the RLS symptoms.[45-47] In contrast, bupropion might alleviate RLS symptoms with its dopamine agonist mechanism.[48] Trazodone also might have a beneficial effect on RLS.[49]

Given the effects of these medications on RLS symptoms, it is important to screen for RLS symptoms before initiating antidepressant therapy. In fact, for a patient with severe RLS and mild depressive symptoms, it is reasonable to treat RLS first to see if an improvement in sleep and energy leads to an improvement of depressive symptoms. When treating depression in patients with severe RLS, clinicians should consider initially trying non-SSRI or non-TCA antidepressants (eg, bupropion). However, there are currently no studies on the comparative efficacy and safety involving bupropion and SSRIs for comorbid depression and RLS.

■ RLS and Other Psychiatric Medications

In the treatment of mood disorders, especially bipolar disorder, the utilization of lithium or anticonvulsants (eg, valproic acid, lamotrigine, or carbamazepine) to stabilize mood is standard practice. In general, it is thought that anticonvulsants associated with pain relief ameliorate RLS symptoms. In fact, gabapentin and carbamazepine have been long considered as second-line agents for the treatment of RLS as double-blind studies reported their efficacy in treating RLS symptoms.[50,51] Valproic acid might be also helpful in reducing RLS symptoms.[52] However, several anecdotal reports of lithium exacerbating PLMS or RLS symptoms exist.[53,54] Therefore, anticonvulsants are considered more "RLS-friendly" than lithium as

12

a mood stabilizer. However, switching lithium to an anticonvulsant as a mood stabilizer should not be undertaken lightly for bipolar disorder patients with RLS regardless of severity of RLS symptoms. Lithium remains the standard as a mood stabilizer in management of bipolar disorder, and a stability of bipolar disorder can be compromised with disastrous results if the switchover destabilizes the mood.

Benzodiazepines and hypnotics are often prescribed to treat insomnia related to psychiatric disorders. Since these medications are not known exacerbate PLMS, their impact on RLS symptoms are assumed to be neutral. Among them, clonazepam is preferred over short-acting benzodiazepines because of its longer half-life. Studies that examined the effect of clonazepam on PLMS and RLS did not find consistent reduction in PLMS; patients instead reported a more restful sleep.[55] Antihistamines are also commonly taken by patients for sleep problems; however, diphenhydramine could exacerbate PLMS and RLS and should be avoided.[56]

Conclusion

RLS is a treatable, common disorder, closely associated with depression and anxiety in both clinics and the community. Given the profound effect of various psychiatric medications on RLS symptoms, the clinicians treating psychiatric disorders in RLS patients should choose medications judiciously to avoid exacerbating RLS symptoms. Evaluation and treatment of RLS in psychiatric practice is poised to become increasingly common as RLS is expected to be elevated to a full diagnosis in DSM-V. However, at the moment, systematic studies on management of psychiatric symptoms and psychiatric medications in RLS patients are lacking. Future studies are warranted to guide clinicians in optimum treatment of psychiatric conditions, particularly depression and anxiety, in RLS patients.

REFERENCES

1. Wittmaack T. *Pathologie und Therapie der Sensibilitäts-Neurosen.* Leipzig, Germany: E Schäfer; 1861:459.

2. Picchietti D, Winkelman JW. Restless legs syndrome, periodic limb movements in sleep, and depression. *Sleep.* 2005;28:891-898.

3. American Psychiatric Association. DSM-5 Development. APA Web site. http://www.dsm5.org/ProposedRevisions/Pages/proposedrevision.aspx?rid=403#. Accessed March 13, 2013.

4. Allen RP, Picchietti D, Hening WA, et al. Restless legs syndrome: diagnostic criteria, special considerations, and epidemiology. A report from the restless legs syndrome diagnosis and epidemiology workshop at the National Institutes of Health. *Sleep Med.* 2003;4:101-109.

5. Robins LN, Helzer JE, Weissman MM, et al. Lifetime prevalence of specific psychiatric disorders in three sites. *Arch Gen Psychiatry.* 1984;41:949-958.

6. Burke KC, Burke JD Jr, Regier DA, Rae DS. Age at onset of selected mental disorders in five community populations. *Arch Gen Psychiatry.* 1990;47:511-518.

7. Berger K, Luedemann J, Trenkwalder C, John U, Kessler C. Sex and the risk of restless legs syndrome in the general population. *Arch Intern Med.* 2004;164:196-202.

8. Walters AS, Hickey K, Maltzman J, et al. A questionnaire study of 138 patients with restless legs syndrome: the 'Night-Walkers' survey. *Neurology.* 1996;46:92-95.

9. Winkelmann J, Muller-Myhsok B, Wittchen HU, et al. Complex segregation analysis of restless legs syndrome provides evidence for an autosomal dominant mode of inheritance in early age at onset families. *Ann Neurol.* 2002;52:297-302.

10. Winkelmann J, Prager M, Lieb R, et al. "Anxietas tibiarum". Depression and anxiety disorders in patients with restless legs syndrome. *J Neurol.* 2005;252:67-71.

11. Lee HB, Hening WA, Allen RP, et al. Restless legs syndrome is associated with DSM IV major depressive disorder and panic disorder in the community. *J Neuropsychiatry Clin Neurosci.* 2007;48:167-169.

12. Cho SJ, Hong JP, Hahm BJ, et al. Restless legs syndrome in a community sample of Korean adults: prevalence, impact on quality of life, and association with DSM-IV psychiatric disorders. *Sleep.* 2009;32(8):1069-1076.

12

13. Cortese S, Konofal E, Lecendreux M, et al. Restless legs syndrome and attention-deficit/hyperactivity disorder: a review of the literature. *Sleep.* 2005;28:1007-1013.

14. Menza MA, Robertson-Hoffman DE, Bonapace AS. Parkinson's disease and anxiety: comorbidity with depression. *Biol Psychiatry.* 1993;34:465-470.

15. Cummings JL. Depression and Parkinson's disease: a review. *Am J Psychiatry.* 1992;149:443-454.

16. Hening WA, Allen RP, Earley CJ, Picchietti DL, Silber MH; Restless Legs Syndrome Task Force of the Standards of Practice Committee of the American Academy of Sleep Medicine. An update on the dopaminergic treatment of restless legs syndrome and periodic limb movement disorder. *Sleep.* 2004;27:560-583.

17. Dunlop BW, Nemeroff CB. The role of dopamine in the pathophysiology of depression. *Arch Gen Psychiatry.* 2007;64:327-337.

18. Feighner JP, Meredith CH, Stern WC, Hendrickson G, Miller LL. A double-blind study of bupropion and placebo in depression. *Am J Psychiatry.* 1984;141:525-529.

19. Goldberg JF, Burdick KE, Endick CJ. Preliminary randomized, double-blind, placebo-controlled trial of pramipexole added to mood stabilizers for treatment-resistant bipolar depression. *Am J Psychiatry.* 2004;161:564-566.

20. Benes H, Mattern W, Peglau I, et al. Ropinirole improves depressive symptoms and restless legs syndrome severity in RLS patients: a multicentre, randomized, placebo-controlled study. *J Neurol.* 2011;258(6):1046-1054.

21. Montagna P, Hornyak M, Ulfberg J, et al.Randomized trial of pramipexole for patients with restless legs syndrome (RLS) and RLS-related impairment of mood. *Sleep Med.* 2011;12(1):34-40.

22. Chervin RD, Archbold KH, Dillon JE, et al. Associations between symptoms of inattention, hyperactivity, restless legs, and periodic leg movements. *Sleep.* 2002;25:213-218.

23. Picchietti D, Allen RP, Walters AS, Davidson JE, Myers A, Ferini-Strambi L. Restless legs syndrome: prevalence and impact in children and adolescents–the Peds REST study. *Pediatrics.* 2007;120(2):253-266.

24. Wagner ML, Walters AS, Fisher BC. Symptoms of attention-deficit/hyperactivity disorder in adults with restless legs syndrome. *Sleep.* 2004;27:1499-1504.

25. Pearson VE, Allen RP, Dean T, Gamaldo CE, Lesage SR, Earley CJ. Cognitive deficits associated with restless legs syndrome (RLS). *Sleep Med.* 2006;7(1):25-30.

26. Fulda S, Beitinger ME, Reppermund S, Winkelmann J, Wetter TC. Short-term attention and verbal fluency is decreased in restless legs syndrome patients. *Mov Disord.* 2010;25(15): 2641-2648.

27. Gamaldo CE, Benbrook AR, Allen RP, Oguntimein O, Earley CJ. A further evaluation of the cognitive deficits associated with restless legs syndrome (RLS). *Sleep Med.* 2008;9(5):500-505.

28. Celle S, Roche F, Kerleroux J, et al. Prevalence and clinical correlates of restless legs syndrome in an elderly French population: the synapse study. *J Gerontol Biol Sci Med Sci.* 2010; 65(2):167-173.

29. Driver-Dunckley E, Connor D, Hentz J, et al. No evidence for cognitive dysfunction or depression in patients with mild restless legs syndrome. *Mov Disord.* 2009;24:1843-1847.

30. Kraus T, Schuld A, Pollmacher T. Periodic leg movements in sleep and restless legs syndrome probably caused by olanzapine. *J Clin Psychopharmacol.* 1999;19:478-479.

31. Wetter TC, Brunner J, Bronisch T. Restless legs syndrome probably induced by risperidone treatment. *Pharmacopsychiatry.* 2002;35:109-111.

32. Pinninti NR, Mago R, Townsend J, Doghramji K. Periodic restless legs syndrome associated with quetiapine use: a case report. *J Clin Psychopharmacol.* 2005;25:617-618.

33. Duggal HS, Mendhekar DN. Clozapine-associated restless legs syndrome. *J Clin Psychopharmacol.* 2007;27:89-90.

34. Montplaisir J, Lorrain D, Godbout R. Restless legs syndrome and periodic leg movements in sleep: the primary role of dopaminergic mechanism. *Eur Neurol.* 1991;31:41-43.

35. Garvey MJ, Tollefson GD. Occurrence of myoclonus in patients treated with cyclic antidepressants. *Arch Gen Psychiatry.* 1987; 44:269-272.

36. Yang C, White DP, Winkelman JW. Antidepressants and periodic leg movements of sleep. *Biol Psychiatry.* 2005;58:510-514.

37. Winkelman JW, James L. Serotonergic antidepressants are associated with REM sleep without atonia. *Sleep.* 2004;27:317-321.

38. Bakshi R. Fluoxetine and restless legs syndrome. *J Neurol Sci.* 1996;142:151-152.

12

39. Sanz-Fuentenebro FJ, Huidobro A, Tejadas-Rivas A. Restless legs syndrome and paroxetine. *Acta Psychiatr Scand*. 1996; 94:482-484.

40. Perroud N, Lazignac C, Baleydier B, Cicotti A, Maris S, Damsa C. Restless legs syndrome induced by citalopram: a psychiatric emergency? *Gen Hosp Psychiatry*. 2007;29:72-74.

41. Hargrave R, Beckley DJ. Restless leg syndrome exacerbated by sertraline. *Psychosomatics*. 1998;39:177-178.

42. Salin-Pascual RJ, Galicia-Polo L, Drucker-Colin R. Sleep changes after 4 consecutive days of venlafaxine administration in normal volunteers. *J Clin Psychiatry*. 1997;58:348-350.

43. Dimmitt SB, Riley GJ. Selective serotonin receptor uptake inhibitors can reduce restless legs symptoms. *Arch Intern Med*. 2000;160:712.

44. Brown LK, Dedrick DL, Doggett JW, Guido PS. Antidepressant medication use and restless legs syndrome in patients presenting with insomnia. *Sleep Med*. 2005;6:443-450.

45. Bahk WM, Pae CU, Chae JH, Jun TY, Kim KS. Mirtazapine may have the propensity for developing a restless legs syndrome? A case report. *Psychiatry Clin Neurosci*. 2002;56:209-210.

46. Teive HA, de Quadros A, Barros FC, Werneck LC. Worsening of autosomal dominant restless legs syndrome after use of mirtazapine: case report. *Arq Neuropsiquiatr*. 2002;60:1025-1029.

47. Agargun MY, Kara H, Ozbek H, Tombul T, Ozer OA. Restless legs syndrome induced by mirtazapine. *J Clin Psychiatry*. 2002;63:1179.

48. Nofzinger EA, Fasiczka A, Berman S, Thase ME. Bupropion SR reduces periodic limb movements associated with arousals from sleep in depressed patients with periodic limb movement disorder. *J Clin Psychiatry*. 2000;61:858-862.

49. Saletu-Zyhlarz GM, Abu-Bakr MH, Anderer P, et al. Insomnia in depression: differences in objective and subjective sleep and awakening quality to normal controls and acute effects of trazodone. *Prog Neuropsychopharmacol Biol Psychiatry*. 2002;26:249-260.

50. Garcia-Borreguero D, Larrosa O, de la Llave Y, Verger K, Masramon X, Hernandez G. Treatment of restless legs syndrome with gabapentin: a double-blind, cross-over study. *Neurology*. 2002;59:1573-1579.

51. Telstad W, Sørensen O, Larsen S, Lillevold PE, Stensrud P, Nyberg-Hansen R. Treatment of the restless legs syndrome with carbamazepine: a double blind study. *Br Med J (Clin Res Ed)*. 1984;288(6415):444-446.

52. Eisensehr I, Ehrenberg BL, Rogge Solti S, Noachtar S. Treatment of idiopathic restless legs syndrome (RLS) with slow-release valproic acid compared with slow-release levodopa/benserazid. *J Neurol*. 2004;251:579-583.

53. Terao T, Terao M, Yoshimura R, Abe K. Restless legs syndrome induced by lithium. *Biol Psychiatry*. 1991;30:1167-1170.

54. Evidente VG, Caviness JN. Focal cortical transient preceding myoclonus during lithium and tricyclic antidepressant therapy. *Neurology*. 1999;52:211-213.

55. Saletu M, Anderer P, Saletu-Zyhlarz G, et al. Restless legs syndrome (RLS) and periodic limb movement disorder (PLMD): acute placebo-controlled sleep laboratory studies with clonazepam. *Eur Neuropsychopharmacol*. 2001;11:153-161.

56. Allen RP, Lesage S, Earley CJ. Anti-histamines and benzodiazepines exacerbate daytime restless legs syndrome symptoms. *Sleep*. 2005;28:A279.

12

13   Closing Remarks

RLS (or WED) and Primary Care and Specialty Practices

It is our hope that this guide may assist both primary care physicians (PCPs) and specialists to manage diverse patients with RLS (a/k/a Willis-Ekbom Disease or WED). Neurologists and sleep disorder specialists will continue to treat more severe, complex cases of RLS. Also, with the anticipated elevation of RLS to its own diagnostic criteria in DSM-V, we also expect more psychiatrists will be diagnosing and treating RLS. Nevertheless, we expect that PCPs will treat the majority of relatively uncomplicated cases of RLS (or WED) encountered in primary care clinics. There are a number of benefits to treating these patients in primary care practice:

- RLS is a relatively common condition that can be readily diagnosed in the clinic without extensive diagnostic work-up.
- RLS is responsive to therapy and treating these patients can have a strong, positive impact on their lives. In fact, treating RLS is often a gratifying experience for both the patients and physicians because of the speedy relief patients commonly obtain from therapy.
- PCPs who provide longitudinal care are in the best position to diagnose and treat RLS patients.

While we have provided information about complex, treatment-resistant RLS patients and the means of treating those patients in this book, satisfactory management of the majority of RLS sufferers may require as little as a single medication prescribed at a low dose to relieve their suffering that might have escaped medical attention for years.

There are many medical specialties in which patients with RLS symptoms can be encountered (**Table 13**.1). Optimal management of these patients will require that their RLS be appropriately evaluated and treated.

When the diagnosis, severity, and management of RLS symptoms appear too complicated and require interventions with which the PCP (or non-RLS specialist) feels uncomfortable, referral of these patients to RLS-specialists for consultation or further management is appropriate. Neurologists (especially those trained in sleep or movement disorders) and sleep-medicine specialists (who may be neurologists, pulmonologists, or psychiatrists) are often familiar with the evaluation and treatment of RLS. Every sleep center is required to have expertise in diagnosing and managing RLS. However, since every neurologist or sleep-medicine specialist is not necessarily an expert in RLS, it could be useful to identify a local RLS expert by contacting the Restless Legs Syndrome Foundation (http://www.rls.org/). There might be a local RLS support group or contact person listed in the Web site that can provide referral to a local RLS clinician as well.

Trends and Prospects

A major step in the treatment of RLS was the approval of several medications, both in the United States and Europe, during the last decade. The three approved dopamine agonists (pramipexole, ropinirole, and rotigotine) are effective and relatively safe medications for treating patients with this condition. More recently, however, the shorter-acting dopamine agonists, such as pramipexole (Mirapex) and ropinirole (Requip), have been associated with augmentation of RLS symptoms that reduces their long-term benefits. The continuously active dopamine agonist, the rotigotine (Neupro) patch, has shown promise in lower rates of troublesome augmentation than other dopamine agonists, while providing excellent relief for most RLS

TABLE 13.1 — Specialities and Patient Groups Vulnerable to RLS

Obstetricians/gynecologists	Women who are pregnant have increased RLS; women, in general, have a 2-fold increased risk of RLS
Pediatricians	About 25% of familial RLS begins in the pediatric age range; children with attention deficit hyperactivity disorder (ADHD) are at increased risk for RLS
Oncologists/hematologists	Anemia and iron deficiency are related to RLS
Pulmonologists	Often involves sleep medicine, therefore, they must be aware of RLS
Internists/renal specialists	RLS is a major morbidity of dialysis; RLS is associated with hypertension and cardiovascular disease
Psychiatrists	Psychoactive medications aggravate RLS; RLS is associated with anxiety and depression
Endocrinologists	RLS is elevated in patients with diabetes and thyroid disorders
Neurologists	RLS is increased in Parkinson disease, multiple sclerosis, and neuropathy
Rheumatologists	RLS is increased in rheumatoid arthritis and other rheumatic conditions
Surgeons	RLS is increased by dopamine blocking and antihistaminergic medications used for sedation during procedures; RLS is increased in lung and heart transplants

13

patients who had been on rotigotine patch for up to 5 years. With the long-term safety and effectiveness data available, rotigotine is arguably the preferred dopamine agonist choice over other options. Nevertheless, the field awaits a comparative effective trial between rotigotine and other dopamine agonists to provide better clinical evidence.

The approval of gabapentin enacarbil (Horizant) for RLS provides a safe and effective alternative to dopaminergic treatment. This medication affects the alpha-2-delta calcium channel reducing neurotransmitter release particularly for glutamate. Drugs in this class (eg, gabapentin, pregabalin, and gabapentin enacarbil) appear to not cause the long-term problems related to augmentation. Gabapentin enacarbil (Horizant) is long-acting and has shown excellent efficacy and safety in the treatment of RLS. A recent consensus statement on the long-term treatment of RLS by the IRLSSG (available on line at www.IRLSG.org) listed the alpha-2-delta drug (gabapentin enacarbil), along with long-acting dopamine agonists (eg, rotigotine), as the first-line pharmacologic treatment option for RLS, with the shorter-acting dopamine agonists used when appropriate in low doses (with careful monitoring for augmentation).

New medications are likely to become available and approved for the treatment of RLS (or WED). Opioids, for example, have long been considered useful in treating RLS, but none have been approved as safe and effective for the treatment of RLS. For example, a low-dose methadone was reported to be effective for over several years in severe cases of RLS.[1] It also seems likely, given the interaction between adenosine and dopamine receptors, that some adenosine receptor medications may be developed for RLS. Another potential future advancement in RLS treatment would be the development of an effective delivery system to ameliorate the apparent brain iron deficiency in RLS. It seems likely that a more efficient delivery system than an oral supplementation of iron may be developed to treat RLS. Certainly some formulation of IV iron therapy could be proven safe and effective for RLS treatment in the future.

Finally, as we learn more about the pathophysiology of RLS and its biological substrates (particularly in relation to brain iron[2] and genetics[3-5]), it is likely we will develop ways to decrease the risk of developing RLS, as well as develop preventive strategies or alter the disease course. Accomplishing these goals will help reduce suffering for a significant percentage of adults and reduce societal costs associated with RLS.

The developments in clinical and basic science have debunked the myth of RLS as a product of disease mongering. The clinical significance of RLS[6] is unquestionable, but clinicians should be judicious in providing careful evaluation and treatment of RLS sufferers. We certainly hope that our readers find that diagnosing and treating RLS becomes a routine and rewarding aspect of their practice.

13

REFERENCES

1. Silver N, Allen RP, Senerth J, Earley CJ. A 10-year, longitudinal assessment of dopamine agonists and methadone in the treatment of restless legs syndrome. *Sleep Med.* 2011; 12(5):440-444.

2. Allen RP, Earley CJ. The role of iron in restless legs syndrome. *Mov Disord.* 2007;22(suppl 18):S440-S448.

3. Winkelmann J, Schormair B, Lichtner P, et al. Genome-wide association study in restless legs syndrome identifies common variants in three genomic regions. *Nat Genet.* 2007;39(8):1000-1006.

4. Winkelmann J, Lichtner P, Schormair B, et al. Variants in the neuronal nitric oxide synthase (nNOS, NOS1) gene are associated with restless legs syndrome. *Mov Disord.* 2008;23(3):350-358.

5. Stefansson H, Rye DB, Hicks A, et al. A genetic risk factor for periodic limb movements in sleep. *N Engl J Med.* 2007;357(7): 639-647.

6. Hening WA, Allen RP, Chaudhuri KR, et al. Clinical significance of RLS. *Mov Disord.* 2007;22(suppl 18):S395-S400.

Appendix A

The International Restless Legs Syndrome (IRLS) Study Group Rating Scale

The subject is asked, "In the past week…"*

1. Overall, how would you rate the RLS discomfort in your legs or arms?
   4—Very severe
   3—Severe
   2—Moderate
   1—Mild
   0—None

2. Overall, how would you rate the need to move around because of your RLS symptoms?
   4—Very severe
   3—Severe
   2—Moderate
   1—Mild
   0—None

3. Overall, how much relief of your RLS arm or leg discomfort did you get from moving around?
   4—No relief
   3—Mild relief
   2—Moderate relief
   1—Either complete or almost complete relief
   0—No RLS symptoms to be relieved

14

---

* It may be helpful to repeat the time frame with each question. One week is the time period most used for clinical trials; the original validation study used 2 weeks as the time period. Other time periods are possible, but if <1 week, question 7 may not work.

4. How severe was your sleep disturbance due to your RLS symptoms?

4—Very severe

3—Severe

2—Moderate

1—Mild

0—None

5. How severe was your tiredness or sleepiness during the day due to your RLS symptoms?

4—Very severe

3—Severe

2—Moderate

1—Mild

0—None

6. How severe was your RLS as a whole?

4—Very severe

3—Severe

2—Moderate

1—Mild

0—None

7. How often did you experience RLS symptoms?

4—Very often (6-7 days in 1 week)

3—Often (4-5 days in 1 week)

2—Sometimes (2-3 days in 1 week)

1—Occasionally (1 day in 1 week)

0—Never

8. When you had RLS symptoms, how severe were they on an average?

4—Very severe (8 h or more per 24 h)

3—Severe (3-8 h per 24 h)

2—Moderate (1-3 h per 24 h)

1—Mild (less than 1 h per 24 h)

0—None

9. Overall, how severe was the impact of your RLS symptoms on your ability to carry out your daily affairs, for example, carrying out a satisfactory family, home, social, school or work life?

4—Very severe
3—Severe
2—Moderate
1—Mild
0—None

10. How severe was your mood disturbance due to your RLS symptoms—for example, angry, depressed, sad, anxious, or irritable?
4—Very severe
3—Severe
2—Moderate
1—Mild
0—None

Each question is scored from 0 for no problem or RLS or symptoms to 4 for very severe. As a rough guide, the overall score can be divided into different levels of severity:

0	No RLS
1-10	Mild RLS
11-20	Moderate RLS
21-30	Severe RLS
31-40	Very severe RLS

The scale can provide a single factor involving all of the items summed.[1] It is also possible to divide the scale into a symptom factor (sum of items 1, 2, 4, 6, 7, 8) and an impact factor (sum of items 5, 9, 10).[2,3]

14

The IRLS is not a diagnostic instrument. It should only be used after the diagnosis of RLS is confirmed. Since the questions all refer to RLS, the patient must be aware of the RLS symptoms and should be able to distinguish them from other feelings or problems.

FIGURE A.1 — Augmentation Severity Rating Scale (ASRS)

Baseline Examination

Instructions: The examiner will ask the patient the following questions. The examiner will read the questions, explain the question, assist the patient in finding the answer, and mark the patient's answer on the form. However, it will be the patient's decision to determine which is the final answer.

Item 1 During the past week, at what time did your RLS symptoms usually start? |__|__| : |__|__| 24-hr clock

Please write down the time when the symptoms usually started (eg: 22:45). HH MM

Item 2 During the past week, at any times you were sitting or resting (for example in a car, plane, theatre or watching TV) how soon afterwards did your RLS symptoms usually start?

Please indicate the time it takes for symptoms to start at various times during the day (late morning, early afternoon, late afternoon, evening before taking any RLS medication).

2a When sitting in the late morning (ie, before noon), your symptoms usually started…

2b When sitting in the early afternoon (ie, 12:00-15:00), your symptoms usually started…

2c When sitting in the late afternoon (ie, 15:00-18:00), your symptoms usually started…

2d When sitting in the evening (after 18:00, before taking the first dose of RLS medication), your symptoms usually started…

- ☐ 0=After a very long time or never
- ☐ 1=After a long time (ie, after about an hour)

- □ 2 = After a moderate amount of time (i.e., after about half an hour)
- □ 3 = After a short time (ie, within a few minutes)
- □ 4 = Immediately or almost immediately
- □ -9 = Did not sit or rest in the morning over the last week

Item 3 During the past week, what parts of your body are usually affected by RLS symptoms?

Please let the patient shade in the figure the portions of his/her body affected by RLS symptoms and choose the corresponding score:

Count 1 point for any of the 8 areas:
- lower legs + feet—left/right
- upper legs—left/right
- arms + hands—left/right
- lower trunk
- upper trunk + head

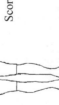

Score (0 - 8)

14

Continued

FIGURE A.1 — Continued

On Treatment Evaluation

Instructions: The examiner will ask the patient the following questions. The examiner will read the questions, explain the question, assist the patient in finding the answer, and mark the patient's answer on the form. However, it will be the patient's decision to determine which is the final answer.

Item 1 During the past week, at what time did your RLS symptoms usually start?

|__|__| : |__|__| 24-hr clock
HH   MM

Please write down the time when the symptoms usually started (eg: 22:45).

Item 2 During the past week, at any times you were sitting or resting (for example in a car, plane, theatre or watching TV) how soon afterwards did your RLS symptoms usually start?

Please indicate the time it takes for symptoms to start at various times during the day (late morning, early afternoon, late afternoon, evening before taking any RLS medication).

2a When sitting in the late morning (ie, before noon), your symptoms usually started…

2b When sitting in the early afternoon (ie, 12:00-15:00), your symptoms usually started…

2c When sitting in the late afternoon (ie, 15:00-18:00), your symptoms usually started…

2d When sitting in the evening (after 18:00, before taking the first dose of RLS medication), your symptoms usually started…

    ☐   0 = After a very long time or never

    ☐   1 = After a long time (ie, after about an hour)

□ 2 = After a moderate amount of time (i.e., after about half an hour)

□ 3 = After a short time (ie, within a few minutes)

□ 4 = Immediately or almost immediately.

□ -9 = Did not sit or rest in the morning over the last week

Item 3 During the past week, what parts of your body are usually affected by RLS symptoms?

Please let the patient shade in the figure the portions of his/her body affected by RLS symptoms and choose the corresponding score:

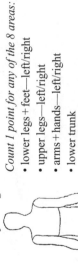

Count 1 point for any of the 8 areas:
- lower legs + feet—left/right
- upper legs—left/right
- arms + hands—left/right
- lower trunk
- upper trunk + head

Score (0 - 8)

14

Continued

FIGURE A.1 — Continued

Evaluation

I. Item 1: Earlier Onset of RLS Symptoms

Please copy the value of item 1 according to the baseline and post-treatment evaluation sheets.

A. at baseline (hrs)

B. at present (hrs)

C. Provide the time difference between A and B (eg. A−B=20:45−17:30=3:15).

Please transform the value of C into a score according to the following scale (in case B>A, mark 0!):

<1 hr: 0
1-<2 hr: 1
2-<3 hr: 2
3-<4 hr: 3
4-<5 hr: 4
5-<6 hr: 5
6-<7 hr: 6
7-<8 hr: 7
≥8 hr: 8

↑

II. Item 3: Usual Latency After Which RLS Symptoms Started When Patient Is at Rest[a]

	2a	2b	2c	2d

A. at baseline

B. at present

C. enter (B − A) (minimal value is 0!): →

Total of the two largest scores (**2a-2d**, maximum = 8)

[a1)] Calculate for each time period and use the two largest values.

2) Code "-9" values as missing and do not calculate a value for this item.

III. Item 4: Spreading of RLS Symptoms:

A. at baseline

B. at present

C. enter (**B − A**) (minimal value is 0!): →

ASRS - Total Score

Please add: **I + II + III**   (maximum = 24) →

14

REFERENCES

1. Walters AS, LeBrocq C, Dhar A, et al; International Restless Legs Syndrome Study Group. Validation of the International Restless Legs Syndrome Study Group rating scale for restless legs syndrome. *Sleep Med*. 2003;4(2):121-132.

2. Allen RP, Kushida CA, Atkinson MJ; RLS QoL Consortium. Factor analysis of the International Restless Legs Syndrome Study Group's scale for restless legs severity. *Sleep Med*. 2003;4(2):133-135.

3. Abetz L, Arbuckle R, Allen RP, et al. The reliability, validity and responsiveness of the International Restless Legs Syndrome Study Group rating scale and subscales in a clinical-trial setting. *Sleep Med*. 2006;7(4):340-349.

Appendix B

Books, Web Information, Patient Organizations, and Resources for RLS

Books

Buchfuhrer MJ, Hening WA, Kushida CA. *Restless Legs Syndrome; Coping With Your Sleepless Nights*. New York: Demos Medical Publishing; 2006.

   Written for patients, this book covers the full spectrum of RLS topics including diagnosis, clinical features, pathogenesis, history, treatment (both drug and nondrug), relationships, disability, and children. With its many useful resources and detailed descriptions on how to treat many difficult RLS situations, it is also suitable reading for primary care physicians.

Chaudhuri KR, Odin P, Olanow CW. *Restless Legs Syndrome*. New York: Taylor & Francis; 2004.

   This is the first professional-level book written on RLS. Written by a panel of experts, *Restless Legs Syndrome* focuses on the diagnosis and management of RLS. The authors discuss the epidemiology of RLS, pathophysiology, clinical associations, and clinical features. They explore how to diagnose the many different types of people who present with this disorder. It includes discussions of the wide range of treatment options available in order to give clinicians the information they need to formulate appropriate pharmacologic or nonpharmacologic therapeutic regimens.

15

Gunzel J. *Restless Legs Syndrome: The RLS Rebel's Survival Guide. Tucson, AZ:* Wheatmark, Inc; 2006.

This book describes the RLS Rebel Program, an outline that helps RLSers (people with RLS) organize their fight against RLS and achieve maximum results from any combination of RLS treatments. When treatments include use of prescription drugs, the RLS Rebel Program becomes the ultimate complementary-medicine approach to RLS. The book includes six steps for reducing aggravating variables, suggestions for developing and using a "bag of tricks" approach, tips for better communication with medical professionals, advice to supporters of RLSers, suggestions for using the RLS Rebel Program in children, and information about dealing with RLS on long trips and in other special situations.

Ondo WG. *Restless Leg Syndrome (Neurological Disease and Therapy).* New York: Informa Healthcare/Taylor & Francis; 2006.

This book, edited by William Ondo, is an authoritative and comprehensive guide on RLS. It examines the pathogenesis, diagnosis, and treatment the disorder. Ranging from basic science to therapeutics, this book analyzes the many new and emerging medications impacting the management of this disorder and strives to address the explosion of research in the field.

Wilson VN, Walters AS, eds. *Sleep Thief, Restless Legs Syndrome.* Orange Park, FL: Galaxy Books Inc; 1996.

This is the first book published on RLS. Written by one of the founders of the RLS Foundation, it contains both a layperson's perspective and professional essays from a variety of medical experts.

Yoakum R. *Restless Legs Syndrome: Relief and Hope for Sleepless Victims of a Hidden Epidemic.* New York: Simon & Schuster; 2006.

This book details the reality of RLS and its problems, as well as reviewing coping, therapy, and the science of RLS. It brings alive the real suffering of the patient with severe

RLS and includes a multitude of individual testimonies. The author is a former member of the Board of Directors of the RLS Foundation and author of the historical article on RLS published in *Modern Maturity* in 1994. He prepared this volume in consultation with a variety of RLS experts, including members of the RLSF Medical Advisory Board.

The Official Patient's Sourcebook on Restless Leg Syndrome. San Diego, CA: Icon Health Publications; 2002.
This volume draws from public, academic, government, and peer-reviewed research; provides guidance on how to obtain free-of-charge, primary research results as well as more detailed information via the Internet. Ebook and electronic versions of this sourcebook are fully interactive with each of the Internet sites mentioned.

Web-Based Information

American Academy of Sleep Medicine (AASM)
www.aasmnet.org
The American Academy of Sleep Medicine is the premier organization devoted to the advancement of sleep medicine and sleep-related research. It also serves as the key resource for public and professional education on sleep disorders. The AASM's educational website is at www. sleepeducation.com (which also includes patient information and on-line forums), and individuals with sleep problems can locate the sleep center nearest to them at www.sleepcenters.org.

Bandolier Website
www.medicine.ox.ac.uk/bandolier

15

Bandolier is a publishing company that has print and Internet versions of medical articles. By typing RLS in its search box, you will find reviews of many articles on RLS.

Johns Hopkins Center for RLS

http://www.hopkinsmedicine.org/neurology_neurosurgery/
specialty_areas/restless-legs-syndrome

This website has educational and research information
on RLS. Johns Hopkins is the most active center doing
research on the role of dopamine and iron in RLS.

National Institutes of Health (NIH)

www.nih.gov

The NIH, a part of the US Department of Health and
Human Services, is the primary federal agency conducting
and supporting medical research. Many other organizations
make up the NIH, covering different health specialties.
Two of these offer valuable information on RLS:

National Institute of Neurological Disorders and Stroke
(NINDS) www.ninds.nih.gov

The NINDS website contains a wealth of information
on neurologic disorders. The site contains a Restless
Legs Syndrome Information Page (*www.ninds.nih.gov/
disorders/restless_legs/restless_legs.htm#What_is*) and
a Restless Legs Syndrome Fact Sheet Page (*www.ninds.
nih.gov/disorders/restless_legs/vdetail_restless_legs.htm*).

The National Heart, Lung, and Blood Institute (NHLBI)
www.nhlbi.nih.gov/index.htm

The NHLBI has a sleep section (*www.nhlbi.nih.gov/health/
public/sleep/rls.htm*) where you can download or order a
free 4-page pamphlet Fact Sheet on RLS. They also have
another Web page (*www.nhlbi.nih.gov/health/prof/sleep/
rls_gde.htm*) where you can download or order a free
hard copy of this 16-page document called *Restless Legs
Syndrome: Detection and Management in Primary Care.*

Patient Organizations and Web Resources

RLS Foundation

www.rls.org

The RLS Foundation is the international nonprofit RLS organization based in Rochester, Minnesota, that has advocated for and helped RLS patients since its inception in 1992. Their website contains information for patients on every aspect of RLS, including a list of doctors who treat RLS. Brochures can be obtained on many RLS topics and they publish a quarterly newsletter, *NightWalkers.* They also supply a medical-alert card that details the drugs that patients should avoid.

In addition to supporting patients, the RLS Foundation helps doctors with research grants for RLS, provides a quarterly scientific bulletin, brochures, and other information to aid in the treatment and understanding of this disorder. Physicians can join a list of medical providers who treat RLS, which may increase their access to RLS patients.

■ *RLS Foundation Pamphlets and Videos*
   Living with RLS
   Surgery and RLS
   Depression and RLS
   Pregnancy and RLS
   Children and RLS
   Medical Bulletin (reviews RLS treatment)
   RLS Scientific Bulletin (reviews RLS research and new treatments)
   RLS: Detection & Management in Primary Care (NIH document)
   Understanding & Diagnosing RLS (video)

The Foundation hosts a forum and chat room where RLS patients can discuss their experiences with others. In addition, it sponsors support groups all over the world, trains support group leaders, and gives financial and educational help.

15

321

Currently there are over 100 support groups in the United States and Canada and several international support groups that work in cooperation with the RLS Foundation. These support groups can be invaluable for patients in many ways. As noted, they help decrease the isolation that RLS sufferers feel and validate that they do indeed have a real disease that is no laughing matter. They can learn about which local doctors are adept at treating RLS, non-pharmacologic therapies (eg, stretches or exercises) that may be beneficial, new drug treatments that are available, and other educational issues. Support groups can also be a forum for patients to share their bad times and successes battling their "tortured limbs." Every patient who has significant RLS is encouraged to join a local support group. If there is not one in their area, encourage the patient to start one (the RLS Foundation will help in doing so).

For patients who are too far from one of the support groups or who do not have the mobility to travel, there are internet support groups and chat/forums that can fulfill this need. Following is a list of these internet sites.

Brain Talk Communities
http://www.braintalkcommunities.org/

Cyberspace RLS Support Group
http://health.groups.yahoo.com/group/rlssupport/

HealthBoard.com
www.healthboards.com

RLS-PLMD at Yahoo Groups
http://health.groups.yahoo.com/group/RLS_PLMD

National Sleep Foundation
www.sleepfoundation.org
The National Sleep Foundation has a wealth of sleep information and an RLS article reviewed by Richard Allen, PhD and Merrill M. Mitler, PhD.

Talk About Sleep

www.talkaboutsleep.com

This site covers many sleep topics, including RLS. It also has chat rooms and message boards on RLS/PLMD topics.

The RLS Rebel Website

www.rlsrebel.com

This site is written by Jill Gunzel, aka the "RLS Rebel," and is a must read for all people with RLS. Jill has suffered from RLS for over 40 years and has a innovative approach for treating RLS. Included are many novel tricks to combat RLS symptoms.

The Southern California RLS Support Group

www.rlshelp.org

This site contains detailed information about the drugs used for RLS and has pages of letters from people all over the world with medical replies from an author of this book, Mark J. Buchfuhrer, MD. Patients can download free medical-alert cards from this site.

15

16 Abbreviations/Acronyms

AASM	American Academy of Sleep Medicine
ACT	activity accounts (measure of motor restlessness)
ADHD	attention deficit/hyperactivity disorder
ANCOVA	analysis of covariance
ASRS	Augmentation Severity Rating Scale
Biceps Brac	biceps brachii
BMI	body mass index
BUN	blood urea nitrogen
CAM	complementary and alternative medicine
cAMP	cyclic adenosine monophosphate
CBC	complete blood count
CHD	coronary heart disease
CGI	Clinical Global Impressions (scale)
CGI-1	Clinical Global Impressions score (item 1)
CI	confidence interval
CNS	central nervous system
COMT	catechol-0-methyl transferase
COPD	chronic obstructive pulmonary disease
CSF	cerebrospinal fluid
CT	computed tomography
DSM	Diagnostic and Statistical Manual of Mental Disorders
ECG	electrocardiogram
EFNS	European Federation of Neurological Sciences
EMG	electromyelogram
EOG	electrooculogram
ESRD	end-stage renal disease
FDA	Food and Drug Administration
fMRI	functional magnetic resonance imaging
GABA	gamma-aminobutyric acid

HTDI	Hopkins Telephone Diagnostic Interview
ICD	impulse control disorder
ICSD	International Classification of Sleep Disorders
IRLS	International Restless Legs Syndrome Rating Scale
IRLSSG	International Restless Legs Syndrome Study Group
JHRLSS	Johns Hopkins Restless Legs Scale
KECA-R	Korean Epidemiologic Catchment Area study Replication
LOCF	last observation carried forward
MDD	major depressive disorder
MOS	Medical Outcomes Scales for Sleep
MRI	magnetic resonance imaging
mSIT	modified SIT to allow restless movements to alleviate symptoms
MSLT	Multiple Sleep Latency Test
Mylo	mylohyoideus
NCCAM	National Center for Complementary and Alternative Medicine
NIH	National Institutes of Health
NOS	nitrogen oxide synthetase
NREM	non-rapid eye movement (sleep)
OR	odds ratio
OTC	over the counter
PCP	primary care physician
PD	Parkinson's disease
PET	positron emission tomography
Plethysm	plethysmogram
PLM	periodic limb movement(s)
PLMAI	periodic limb movement arousal index
PLMD	periodic limb movement disorder
PLMI	periodic limb movement index
PLMS	periodic limb movement(s) in sleep
PLMSAI	periodic limb movement(s) during sleep arousal index
PLMW	periodic limb movement(s) in wake
prn	as needed
PSG	polysomnography
QOL	quality of life
RBD	REM behavior disorder
REM	rapid eye movement (sleep)

REST	RLS Epidemiology, Symptoms, and Treatment [study]
RiBECA	RLS in Baltimore Epidemiologic Catchment Area
RLS	restless legs syndrome
RLS-DI	Restless legs syndrome diagnostic index
RON	oronasal respirogram
RR	relative risk
RTA	thoraco-abdominal respirogram
SaO_2	oxygen saturation
SBJ	subjective leg discomfort
SF-36	Short Form 36 Health Survey
SIT	suggested immobilization test
SNRI	serotonin-norepinephrine reuptake inhibitor
SNSRI	selective norepinephrine and serotonin reuptake inhibitor
SPECT	single-photon emission computed tomography
SSRI	selective serotonin reuptake inhibitor
System art press	systemic arterial pressure
TCA	tricyclic antidepressant
Tib. ant.	tibialis anterior
TIBC	total iron-binding capacity
TREAT	Therapy with Ropinirole: Efficacy and Tolerability
UARS	upper airway resistance syndrome
VAS	visual analogue scale
WED	Willis-Ekbom Disease

16

INDEX

Note: RLS is the abbreviation for Restless Legs Syndrome;
WED is for Willis-Ekbom Disease.
Page numbers in *italics* refer to figures.
Page numbers followed by a t indicate tables.

17

17

17

17

17

17

17

17

17

17

17

17

17

17

17

17

17

17

17

17